G000144582

Azmina Govindji BSc Hons RD consultant nutritionist and dietitia and Master Practitioner in Neur Azmina started her early career hospitals (gaining direct experienc eight years as the National Consul ~~~~ Diabetes when she was Chief Dietitian to Diabetes UK. This experience makes her particularly qualified to write this book, as GI is a concept that has been used in diabetes for decades. She now runs her own practice providing dietetic consultancy to the food industry, healthcare professionals, the media and the general public. She sits on various Boards within national organisations such as the British Heart Foundation, Diabetes Research & Wellness Foundation and Black and Ethnic Minorities Diabetes Association. She was Chairperson of the British Dietetic Association (BDA) PR Committee and a member of the BDA Executive Council from 2001–4. She is also a member of the BDA Dietitians in Obesity Management Group UK and the Health Professions Council.

In 2002 Azmina won a National Award for Excellence for outstanding professional achievement, as judged by Professor Kenneth Calman, former Chief Medical Officer to the government.

A regular contributor to *Slim at Home*, *Grazia*, BBC *olive* and numerous other magazines, she also appears on TV and radio and is frequently quoted in the national press as spokesperson to the British Dietetic Association. She is currently resident nutritionist on ITV's *This Morning* and also appears on Channel 5's *The Wright Stuff* and Gordon Ramsay's *The F-Word*. Azmina has worked on two diabetes education videos with GMTV's Dr Hilary Jones and is author of over a dozen books, including the best-selling *The Gi Plan* with Nina Puddefoot, *The Diabetes Weight Loss Diet* with TV chef Antony Worrall Thompson and *Think Well to Be Well* with Nina Puddefoot.

She is a great believer in encouraging people to make their own decisions about what they can realistically achieve in their health and lifestyle goals.

Nina Puddefoot has successfully established herself as an independent, global, leading-edge Management Consultant, and director of her own business, over many years. She is qualified as a Master Practitioner and life coach in Neuro-Linguistic Programming (NLP) and holds a Global Certified Trainer and Consultant Certification. She is also on the Editorial Advisory Board for the Diabetes Research & Wellness Foundation.

Nina works with innovative and creative models of thinking within multinational organisations and industries, as well as with individuals, worldwide.

Nina is an author and a regular presenter of public programmes, talks and workshops and has appeared as a guest speaker on The Aurora.

She has featured in a series of programmes about business and health today for television, and works in radio. Other projects include advising the Aga Khan Health Board (UK) and Department of Health on a healthy lifestyle video, writing regular articles and making various contributions to numerous newspapers and popular magazines.

Nina is renowned for her ability to establish relationships quickly with sensitivity and humour, and for enriching and inspiring the lives of others through her passion and support for an individual's empowerment. Ultimately her greatest success is in enabling people to make sustainable and maintainable changes in their life, effortlessly, through her mastery of challenging and supporting the individual during the process.

Azmina Govindji BSc RD and Nina Puddefoot

THE
HOT
BODY
PLAN

LOOK GOOD ...
THE HEALTHY WAY

Vermilion
LONDON

3 5 7 9 10 8 6 4 2

Published in 2007 by Vermilion, an imprint of Ebury Publishing

A Random House Group Company

The Random House Group Limited Reg. No. 954009

Addresses for companies within the Random House Group can be found at www.randomhouse.co.uk

A CIP catalogue record for this book is available from the British Library

The Random House Group Limited makes every effort to ensure that the papers used in our books are made from trees that have been legally sourced from well-managed and credibly certified forests. Our paper procurement policy can be found on www.randomhouse.co.uk

Printed and bound in Great Britain by Cox & Wyman

Designed and set by seagulls.net

ISBN 9780091910525

Copies are available at special rates for bulk orders. Contact the sales development team on 020 7840 8487 for more information.

To buy books by your favourite authors and register for offers, visit www.rbooks.co.uk

The advice offered in this book is not intended to be a substitute for the advice and counsel of your personal physician. Always consult a medical practitioner before embarking on a diet, or a course of exercise. Neither the authors nor the publisher can be held responsible for any loss or claim arising out of the use, or misuse, of the suggestions made, or the failure to take medical advice.

Dedicated to...

The beautiful children in my life: Bizhan, Shazia, Haris, Kamil, Arisha, Ziyana, Aly and Khalil. Children offer an innocent perspective which helps to lighten any adversity. These exceptional young people radiate love and laughter and it is this lightness that reminds me of how everything is a blessing; it just depends on how you look at it.

Azmina

Children and animals have so much to teach us. There's the unconditional love, the stumble or fall which simply means get up and try again and the fun and laughter of being in the now, to name but a few!

For this reason, I am taking this special opportunity to mention my godsons, Harry and Jack Biggs. And, a thank you to their parents, my very dear friends Clare and Paul, for the part they played in bringing them into the world!

And, to all the animal lovers out there, especially my close-knit riding-stable friends, too many to mention!

Nina

CONTENTS

ACKNOWLEDGEMENTS

So many people are involved when a new book gets published – it isn't just about the authors. We would like to thank the special people who have guided us since our very first publication, those who have helped bring this book to life, and friends and family who continually help us to review and refine our work. There are too many to mention, but a handful deserve singling out here:

Expert dietitians, researchers and academics who have offered their support in all our books.

Sue Potter, registered dietitian, for providing an expert critique on dietary aspects of this book.

Smita Ganatra, registered dietitian, Brent Primary Care Trust, for general dietary input.

Our *Hot Body Plan* testers who have tried the Plan and helped to address practical issues before publication – Felicity, Nafisha, Marta, Karima, Lorraine, Sarah, Zohra, Nigel, Sue, Mary, Jaz, Lucy, John and Debbie, and Shairoz for her delicious salsa recipe.

Hard-working student dietitians at King's College, London University for technical assistance – Sasha Watkins and Alison Hornby – and Rajni Jumbu, a conscientious nutritionist who recently qualified from Coventry University.

The manufacturers and retailers who provided extensive GI data on their food products.

Companies who have kindly offered equipment for recipe development – Kenwood, Lakeland, Panasonic, Russell Hobbs, Salton Europe and Kitchen Aid.

Journalists and broadcasters who have believed in our philosophy and helped to promote our publications in the national media.

And, of course, our patient publishers, specifically Julia Kellaway and Caroline Newbury, for their endless support and enthusiasm.

INTRODUCTION:
AZ AND NINA'S GUIDE
TO THE HOT BODY PLAN

et's face it, diets simply don't work. Dieting focuses solely on your body and ignores the most important part of you – your mind! What comes to mind when you hear the word 'diet'? For many, it conjures up food deprivation, too much like hard work, an end to pleasurable eating. Try this. Say to yourself: 'I mustn't eat chocolate. I just can't eat chocolate. I shouldn't go near a chocolate bar.' What are you thinking about? Chocolate, of course! As soon as you say to yourself that you need to avoid a certain food, that food becomes even more desirable. To make the changes you need to make to get the kind of body you want to have, you must make sure your mind is on your side. The brain is an incredibly powerful tool – so why not use it?

If you recognise yourself as a serial dieter or feel that other diets have failed you, then look no further. We offer you here and now, what we believe is the *only* key to success that will guarantee you results. A unique combination of tried-and-tested motivational strategies and filling satisfying meal ideas, intermingled within an achievable exercise plan.

CHANGE YOUR THOUGHTS

Every moment of the day, your feelings, whether you're consciously aware of it or not, come from the pictures you make in your mind and the things you say to yourself. Some people live their lives in a dream-like, unconscious state. Life is something that happens *to* them. Others know the difference and choose to take responsibility for everything that exists in their life. They are willing to make the changes necessary to get what they want.

The feelings that underlie emotional hunger boil down to one thing and that is the negative feelings that you have about yourself. A flatter tum, firmer buns or a few inches off your thighs and waist is something to look forward to. Your body is a temple so, for now, love all you've got by making friends with your 'temple' as it is today. This will support you in getting the body you wish for.

Acceptance without judgement of yourself is a healthy starting place. You are where you are and today is the day you can start to make different choices. Keeping a positive frame of mind is an important step in getting your mind on your side. And what better way, than reminding yourself of all the great people and things that already exist in your life?

Ask yourself the following questions as a positive reminder.

✳ What fills me with happiness in my life today and how does that make me feel?
✳ What am I grateful for?
✳ What am I proud about?
✳ Who loves and cares about me and who do I love and care about?

* What am I enjoying most in my life?
* What aspects of my body do I like?

CHANGE YOUR THOUGHTS AND YOU CHANGE YOUR WORLD

Could these unhelpful questions be familiar to you?

* Why can't I ever start a diet and stick to it?
* Why do I feel so negative about myself?
* Why does this sort of thing always happen to me?

The mind will always oblige by answering and the answers will be in line with the way in which the questions are being asked – in this case, negatively! For example, answers to the above might be: 'Because I'm a loser!' 'I'm an unattractive lump!' 'I'm an idiot!' All pretty self-loathing, right? All these answers come from the way in which the questions are framed. However, when you ask rich, quality questions of yourself, the answers will match. Apart from anything else, research tells us optimists live longer than pessimists, so learn to look for the positive by asking the question in a positive way and believe that every so-called problem has a solution. Try asking, 'What would be an effortless way in which I can achieve my goal?' 'What do I need to do to succeed?'

Believing there is no such thing as failure, only the chance to learn through your experiences, is a powerful belief. Asking yourself what you can learn from any so-called 'failure' can powerfully change the meaning you give to any event or circumstance, including your experience of past diet efforts.

WHAT YOU FOCUS ON, EXPANDS

The richness of the questions will match the quality of the response your brain usefully searches to give you. As a result, you experience a happier and more resourceful state.

Your positive frame of mind will increase your likelihood of achieving any goal that you set out to accomplish.

Check your thoughts and inner dialogue today. You are the bodyguard of your thinking and ultimately your feelings, which lead to your actions. Remember that who you believe yourself to be will be governed by the choices you make.

WHY THIS DIET IS DIFFERENT

It's different because … it isn't a diet! Dieting is all about avoiding. The Hot Body Plan isn't about avoiding. It's about asking yourself which choice you'd rather make. It's about equipping yourself with a treasure chest of tools and lots of swap lists so that you can choose the food or snack that's just right for you at any given moment. And if you're a party animal, chances are that you'll want to let your hair down. So when you're at a party, this isn't about sitting around with a few carrot sticks on your plate. We will show you how to enjoy your Hot Body Plan with a clear conscience, alcohol included!

These days there is more information and advice on healthy eating than ever before. And yet, we face the increasing possibility of an obesity epidemic. This suggests that all the knowledge and education available is simply not enough unless it is supported first and foremost by getting your mind on your side. You also need to understand that who you believe you want to become, the 'new' you, will be supported by your behaviour, and this includes the healthy food choices that you will make.

YOUR LIMITATIONS ARE YOUR EXPECTATIONS

How do you set about turning possibilities into probabilities? Imagine for a moment that you are an energetic, super fit and healthy person; someone who constantly enforces positive self-talk and generally feels great about themselves and life. Given the choice of a fat, starchy rich cream bun or a red juicy apple, the choice is a no-brainer! Your choice is effortlessly in line with your identity. If you think of yourself as an overweight slob, your choice may well be very different and certainly not consistent.

Just trying to change your behaviour by starting a diet is like pushing a cart uphill. It needs to be supported by your identity. Your identity is the dominant force behind your behaviours. Everything this book offers you will work with this golden key in mind. And the changes you make will be maintained and sustained for as long as you are truly committed. This is the factor that will make the difference to your lifestyle changes, permanently.

CHECK YOUR COMMITMENT

Once you are truly committed to making these life-long sustainable changes to achieve your Hot Body, all sorts of things will occur to help you.

Here's the most powerful checklist of all the major points that will get your mind working with you and supporting your new identity.

CHECK ME OUT!

Where do you truly feel you are right now? The following point-ers will give you a realistic indication of what you particularly need to focus your attention on *before* you begin your new healthy eating lifestyle change.

WRITE DOWN YOUR SPECIFIC GOAL

For example: I choose to fit comfortably into my new size 'x' party dress by 'y' date. Keep it realistic – dropping from a size 14 to a size 10 in two weeks is unlikely and unsafe. Rate yourself on the scale of 1–5 as to how committed you are. If your commit-ment rating is below 5, ask yourself what you would need to do to get up to the maximum.

Is there anyone who could support you? Someone who has already achieved what you are aiming for, a role model?

Could you recruit an exercise buddy? Someone who'll encour-age you, have a laugh with you and help you stay motivated?

What else? Make a list. Include any additional support that you would like from friends or family.

Now make a list of all the *benefits* that would come from achieving this. Think ahead to how you will celebrate your success and write down a reward, too.

MY GOAL IS:

THE BENEFITS TO ME IN ACHIEVING THIS ARE:

MY REWARD IS:

YOUR MIND IS A POWERFUL TOOL – USE IT WISELY

Furthermore, your mind doesn't easily know the difference between what's real and what's imagined. By giving it a full-on emotional experience by using all your senses, it will believe what it experiences. For example, when you are completely engrossed in a good thriller, you may find yourself seeing, hearing and feeling as if you are there for real. Perhaps you start to hold your breath as you read and maybe your palms start to sweat, too? This helps to explain why we can become so engrossed in reading. Your imagination is more powerful than your willpower. Give your mind a convincing experience of the new, 'Hot Bodied', you. To do this, you may choose a quiet spot, put 5–10 uninterrupted minutes aside and close your eyes if it helps.

THREE STEPS TO A NEW YOU

STEP ONE

Imagine … yourself on a giant-size cinema screen. See yourself in colour and make the picture bright. This is you, the way you ideally wish to be. It's important you put in as much detail as possible. What do you see? See yourself in the little black number, the hot swimming cossie, skinny jeans or equivalent. Notice how great you look. Pay attention to your posture, gestures and facial expressions. See yourself radiating health, energy and confidence. Who else is in the picture with you?

Hear … your positive self-talk and the compliments you are paying yourself now that you've achieved your goal. Notice the way you speak, listen and laugh. Hear the tone, volume and energy in your voice and any other sounds around you. What are others saying to you? What sort of things are they saying to congratulate you on your success?

Feel … the positivity of your achievements and how this enriches your self-image. What is that doing for you? Notice the natural air of confidence and warmth that you exude. Relate this to the daily activity that you now engage in and love. What other activities do you get involved with?

What else do you notice in the new you that makes you so magnetic, attractive and seductive, so that others are drawn to you like bees to a honey pot?

Feel even more inspiration building up in you as you pay closer attention to your movie.

STEP TWO

Now step into the movie and become the new you. Make any adjustments in your thinking, posture and gestures, so that you feel comfortable in your new skin. Relax and enjoy this experience. Take a few minutes to remind yourself of who you are becoming. Now ask yourself these few questions:

* What is truly important to me about succeeding with this goal?
* How is my life positively different?
* What are the benefits and how much more can I accomplish in my life?
* What is the positive effect on others?
* How much happier do I feel?

Do this exercise several times to start with, adding richness and more meaningful and attractive images and sounds each time. Make it *soooooooo* compelling that your mind will be seduced into assisting you in making it happen. Do it daily to reinforce it. Repetition is the key here. You'll be amazed at how effortlessly you'll begin to attract the things that you really want into your life.

As a result of this exercise, commit to one new behaviour that will support your goal and the new you.

Now look back over your list of benefits. What else might you wish to add as a result of this exercise?

STEP THREE

Well, here's one from us. It's a cheeky little suggestion and a powerful one in terms of proving your commitment to your unconscious and conscious brain. Buy yourself that little black number (or equivalent), in the size that would reflect the new you. (Remember, be realistic!) Hang it up somewhere where you are likely to see it regularly. And, put up a photo of how you'd like to look. It could be one from the past. This will act as a daily reminder. Remember we gravitate in the direction of our dominant thoughts. If you lose the recommended half to one kilo (one to two pounds) per week, you could lose three kilos (half a stone) in a month — steady and certainly noticeable.

PAINTING BY NUMBERS

Paint your own blank canvas and design the life you want. Consider all the important aspects of your life. You may wish to include:

NUMBER ONE: *Identity/self-image*

* What are the five qualities that you would choose to enhance your identity?
* How many of these do you already have?

✳ What would you need to do to develop these?

✳ Write down at least one supporting behaviour per quality that will help you in attaining these characteristics. For example, saying 'thank you' when someone pays you a compliment without trying to justify it.

NUMBER TWO: *Health and fitness*

✳ What is your goal for health and fitness?

✳ What activity could you build into your daily life that would effortlessly fit with your lifestyle and/or what adjustments would you need to make so as you can consistently achieve this?

NUMBER THREE: *Spiritual development*

✳ In which ways could you nurture and nourish yourself?

✳ Consider treatments such as massage, or give yourself 'me' time, when you can find some silent space to simply be, and reconnect with nature by walking in the woods, mountains, by the sea or watching a sunrise or sunset.

When you get a sense of where you most need to make some changes, decide on some tangible and realistic goals within a time frame and write them down.

Examples of the above are:

✳ I am walking 10,000 steps a day (measured by a step counter).

✳ I am putting 20 minutes aside daily to take time out with myself.

✳ I consciously look for the good and beauty in everyone I meet.

WHAT'S SO SPECIAL ABOUT FOOD ON THE HOT BODY PLAN?

Any change in your eating habits needs to be enjoyable if you're going to succeed in the long term. Through our extensive work with people who want to lose weight and keep it off, we have discovered the ideal formula – eat often, eat foods that fill you up and eat for health. Many diets may offer you a quick fix, with impressive weight-loss results in record time. Read the small print and you might find that you're expected to take a range of vitamin and mineral supplements too. Why do you think that might be? It is often because the diet you're being advised to keep to isn't nutritionally balanced and therefore these supplements are needed as a safeguard. The Hot Body Plan has been compiled by highly qualified nutritionists and dietitians and it encompasses good all-round nutrition while being based on sound scientific strategies for weight loss.

Within this, you will notice the plan is based on the glycaemic index, or GI. The concept of GI has been researched for decades, mainly in the field of diabetes and heart disease. Studies have shown that healthy low-GI foods (such as beans, lentils, porridge, pasta, fruit and vegetables, nuts and seeds) can help maintain healthy blood glucose (sugar) levels. This in turn has a beneficial effect on your health and may even prevent conditions such as diabetes and heart disease.

If you're overweight, especially if you carry that weight around your middle, you may be more prone to a condition called *insulin resistance*. Insulin is a hormone that is released by your pancreas in response to the carbohydrates, or 'carbs', you eat. If you eat carbs that make your blood sugar go up very quickly (such as sugary drinks and sweets), this provokes your body to release more insulin. If you do this repeatedly, you could be putting a strain on your pancreas. In time, your body can become more and more resistant to the effect of insulin, and this can make you more prone to conditions such as diabetes, heart disease and metabolic syndrome (sometimes called Syndrome X).

Some carbs will be more slowly digested, they will sit in your gut for longer, and cause much slower rises in your blood glucose. These are your allies in the weight-loss battle – they're the lower-GI foods. They add ammunition (filling food), power (giving you energy for longer because of the way they are digested) and defence (as they help you maintain your new weight and defend you against temptation). And what's more, they taste good! So you're winning all the way.

BE A 'GIPPER' AND FEEL CHIPPER

The Hot Body Plan is based on GiPs (pronounced JiPs) ... a unique system that incorporates GI, portion size and energy or calorie density all rolled into one. In simple terms, by keeping to our GI-based Hot Body Plan, you will automatically be eating healthier foods that are likely to fill you up for longer and that help you get into that party outfit or those skinny jeans. On the following pages you will see tasty meal and menu ideas that are packed with variety and goodness, helping to kick-start your new low-GI, healthy, yet party-hectic, lifestyle.

* Is it about calories? Yes, but you don't need to count them.
* Is it about eating less? No, more like eating the right carbs and enjoying healthy amounts of protein foods that also help keep you full for longer. You might even feel that you're

eating more, as to be a real 'Gipper' you could be eating five times a day. And your plate may be even more packed than before, because you're piling on those filling veggies.

✳ Is it about avoiding fats? No, it's about choosing more of the appropriate types, like nuts and olives, to get you more of the results that you really want.

✳ Is it about going hungry? No, this is the best news of all. Research suggests that low-GI foods, because they are slowly digested, can help prevent hunger pangs.

✳ Will I feel light-headed as I start to eat less? No, remember you're not eating less! In fact, you might be surprised at just how much food is on your plate. Because GI is based on how foods affect your blood sugar levels, choosing to eat the GiP way will help to keep your blood sugar levels slow and steady. This in turn helps provide mental alertness so that you feel energised throughout the day.

✳ Is it a low carb diet? No, it's more of a slow carb diet. Low carb diets do help you to lose weight quickly, but you may find you fall into the common pitfalls of rapid weight-loss diets. Some people do find that they have headaches and lightheadedness on very low carb diets, and missing out on fruit and vegetables and other important carbs can put you at risk of nutritional deficiencies in the long term. Also, eating fewer carbs and lots of protein isn't appropriate for good health. The Hot Body Plan allows you to still enjoy your bread and potatoes – it simply shows you which types are best to give you a lower 'glycaemic effect'.

✳ Why is the choice of carbs important? The glycaemic concept is about the effect of the *type* of carb on your blood sugar and this has consequences for your health. The GI of a carb reflects whether your blood sugar is likely to go up slowly (low GI) or quickly (high GI). The key to feeling fuller for longer, and healthy weight loss, is to choose slower carbs, that is, carbs that are slowly digested.

However, there's no point in eating low-GI foods if you're going to be shovelling them in at every opportunity. And that's why we created GiP. The GiP way of eating is a unique combination of GI and portion sizes, by keeping an eye on the amount you eat while still allowing you your favourite carbs.

All you need to do to get to that Hot Body is set out here in the sections of this book. You'll find an array of tempting ideas for all your meals and snacks. These have been carefully selected for their nutritional and weight-loss benefits, helping you to achieve that flatter tummy. So enjoy your new meals, your new lifestyle, your new outlook and your new you!

Oh, one more point … We know some people don't seem to like making ink marks in their book. However, just weigh this up – if you fill in the boxes here – the exercise boxes, the other suggested goals in the book – you have a powerful reminder of where you are going. If you know where you're going, you're more likely to get there. After all, whose Hot Body is this about? Enjoy the book and doodle away!

AND FINALLY…

✳ The GiP system is all about flexibility. You can mix and match foods to make up your favourite meal.

✳ High fibre doesn't necessarily mean low GI, though many high fibre foods are also low GI. It's the way the carbs are digested that counts, and eating more fibre is a good thing.

✳ By simply changing from high-GI foods (say cornflakes) to a low-GI food (say porridge), you are automatically getting the benefits of low-GI eating. Generally, eating more slow release carbs, such as grainy bread and pasta, means you will have less room for the processed fatty foods, such as pies and sausage rolls.

* People from the Indian sub-continent tend to have a higher risk of conditions like diabetes and metabolic syndrome (Syndrome X). Low-GI foods in the right context may help reduce risks. High-GI foods will demand more insulin from you – and this can, over time, lead you to becoming resistant to your own insulin. South Asians are more insulin-resistant than the wider UK population. In short, enjoy low-GI Indian goodies like dahl and basmati rice!

CHAPTER ONE:
THE 5 PER CENT FACTOR

Often when we start a new eating plan, we set ourselves such unachievable targets that it just seems too huge a task and we give up halfway through. However, there is a wealth of research to show that losing just 5 per cent of your body weight gives you enormous benefits. Check these out for starters:

* Reduced blood cholesterol and other blood fats
* Reduced blood pressure
* Less back and joint pain
* Improved self-esteem and confidence
* More balanced blood sugar levels, which can help maintain your energy levels
* Reduced risk of angina
* Less breathlessness
* Better sleep

HOW TO ASSESS YOUR 5 PER CENT FACTOR

Here's a quick way of determining how much weight you need to lose to get these benefits.

✳ Work out your weight in kilograms (or pounds): for example, 70 kg (150 lb).

✳ Move the decimal place one space to the left, in this case to get 7 kg (15 lb). This is 10 per cent of your weight.

✳ Now halve that amount to give you 5 per cent – that's 3.5 kg (around 7 lb).

You can see that 5 per cent is a really sensible target for you. And if you don't believe us, check out the science at the back of the book.

> 🐾 *Set small goals so that you overachieve and feel great when you do*

GET YOUR MIND ON YOUR SIDE

Getting your mind working with you to support your goals is the key to success. Why? Because you need to think like a slim, trim, healthy, energetic person in order to act like one. All your actions and the choices that you make in your life, including the foods you eat, the amount of exercise you take and the way in which you nurture and nourish yourself is governed through your identity.

CHECK ME OUT

So stop dieting (or don't begin!). Each time you reach for something, go through our *check-me-out* tips:

TIP 1: *Check your hunger*
How hungry are you right now? Could it be emotional hunger? Are you eating just because you see food, or because of the

time, or because you're bored? Use this chart to help you tune in to your own appetite and fullness (satiety) cues. Simply circle the appropriate feeling. As you become more aware of how hungry or full you are, you will be able to resist temptation just because something is in front of you.

Starving   **Pretty hungry**   **Satisfied**   **Full**   **Pigged out!**

TIP 2: *Check it's what you really want*
Is this food going to get you closer to your goals? What do you need to be thinking right now to help you make the best choice? If you go for it, how will you feel soon after? What will you choose?

TIP 3: *Check if you're full*
It's okay to leave something on your plate.

GET INTO THE HABIT OF ASKING YOURSELF 'AM I REALLY HUNGRY?'

Think about your response on a scale of 1 (not hungry) to 10 (starving hungry). You'll be amazed how often you eat when you are scoring only 2 or 3. Whenever you give yourself a low *hunger* score, make a note of what's going on around you, your thoughts and feelings at the time – committing this to paper helps bring the *real* factors for eating to the front of your consciousness. Although we shouldn't eat when we're not hungry, we shouldn't let our hunger levels get to a 9 or 10 either. By leaving long periods between meals and getting ravenously hungry, we're likely to end up overeating.

Whenever you catch yourself feeling tempted by something naughty but nice, another glass of alcohol, missing out your daily activity, or anything else that would fit here, *press the pause button* and ask yourself this all important question:

Is what I am about to do right now going to take me nearer to my goal or not?

If not, choose again. Remind yourself of all the benefits that you wrote down previously. If they are powerful enough, you will make a different choice in that moment that will continue to support your overall goal. It may be useful to make a list of distractions that would work well for you, which you could fall back on. For example:

At a party, to stop automatically reaching for another glass of wine, drink a glass of water. Get up and get dancing. As part of the new, more confident you, go chat to a stranger. It could be the start of a beautiful friendship! For more ideas, see pages 119–24.

At work, muster the energy to deliver a message, some mail or go over and have a conversation with a colleague, which may also mean using the stairs. Make the phone call that you've been putting off. Use your lunch break to get out into the fresh air and take a walk. Carry your weather with you – dull on the outside, sunny on the inside!

> ❧ *'Today, I embrace fresh air, it is a valuable part of my life, but it wasn't always the case. I have been known in days gone by, to drive around three times just so as I could park right outside somewhere! And, don't get me wrong, some days the temptation still lingers!'*

AND FINALLY...

✳ Studies suggest that people who record their progress or what they are eating tend to have better results.

✳ Just 5–10 per cent weight loss can give you significant health benefits.

✳ Low-GI eating is healthy for the whole family, and cooking family meals with emphasis on natural rather than processed foods makes good overall sense.

✳ Try the 20-minute rule. If you're hungry, have some water and do something to distract yourself for 20 minutes. If you still feel hungry, then you probably are! At that point, choose either a GiP-free snack or one of the snacks that are on your menu plan, regardless of the time of day.

✳ The biggest mistake you can make on this diet is not to eat. Missing a meal will actually be counterproductive, so even if you don't feel up to it, try to have regular meals.

✳ Try our light-hearted assessment in the next chapter, designed to give you an idea of where you could pay more attention in order to live the life that you would like.

CHAPTER TWO: YOUR MIND, BODY AND SPIRIT ASSESSMENT

Before you can decide what changes you need to make in terms of mind, body and spirit, you need to find out exactly where you are at the moment. Try to answer the following questions as truthfully as you can. Next, look below at 'The message in the madness – the meaning behind the questions' to find out what your answers say about you (page 27). Finally, at the end of the section, look at the key (see pages 37–9) to see how you scored.

MIND ASSESSMENT

1. *What is your relationship with food?*
   i. Some days, when I'm feeling a tad under the weather or down in the dumps, I reach for the unhealthy snacks.
   ii. The only thing I can't resist is temptation! Food is a comfort to me.
   iii. Mostly, I eat when I'm hungry.

2. *What do you ask yourself when things aren't going your way?*
   i. Why does this always happen to me?
   ii. What should I do instead?
   iii. What should I stop doing?

3. *Think of a goal you have right now. How are you thinking about the goal?*

  i. I am imagining what it would be like to achieve the goal.

  ii. I see a number of barriers and problems that would stop me.

  iii. It is easier for me to identify what I don't want, to start with.

BODY ASSESSMENT

4. *What's your waist measurement?*

Women:	Men:
i. 81–89 cm (32–35 in)	94–102 cm (37–40 in)
ii. 61–81 cm (24–32 in)	69–94 cm (27–37 in)
iii. Over 89 cm (35 in)	Over 102 cm (40 in)

5. *Work out your BMI (Body Mass Index) by measuring your weight (in kilograms) and dividing this by your height (in metres) squared: BMI = weight (kg) ÷ height (m)^2. What is your BMI?*

  i. 20 to 24 (in the okay range).

  ii. Less than 20 or between 25 and 30 (under- or overweight).

  iii. More than 30 (obese).

6. *Your body shape can best be described as …*

  i. Apple shaped.

  ii. Pear shaped.

  iii. In between a pear and an apple shape.

PHYSICAL ASSESSMENT

7. *How do you feel about physical activity?*
   i. A daily dose of activity is actually something that I look forward to.
  ii. I blink regularly, use my arms to lift the glass to my mouth and take the rubbish out weekly ... what more do you want?
 iii. Some days it's hard work trying to motivate myself to get going.

8. *How much exercise do you get on average?*
   i. I get some exercise in the week.
  ii. Once in a blue moon.
 iii. Almost daily.

9. *Which statement best applies to you, regarding physical activity?*
   i. It's been so long, I can't be bothered.
  ii. I would make more of an effort if I had the time.
 iii. Physical activity keeps me upbeat and puts oomph into my day.

FOOD ASSESSMENT

10. *How many colours are there on your plate, on average?*
   i. Two to three colours.
  ii. More than three colours.
 iii. One colour.

11. *Your meal and snack habits tend to be ...*
   i. Three meals a day with two to three light snacks in between.
  ii. Fairly regular, though I often go several hours without eating.
 iii. Very little in the daytime, eat lots in the evenings.

12. Alcohol is like ...

  i. An obsession at times, with copious amounts at weekends.

  ii. A nice companion to my evening meal, about a unit.

  iii. A regular buddy, probably two to three units a day.

13. Which carb do you eat most often?

  i. Rice.

  ii. Pasta.

  iii. Wholemeal bread.

14. Do you eat breakfast ...

  i. Daily?

  ii. Rarely?

  iii. Four to five times a week?

15. When you shop for food, the labels are ...

  i. Just small print, I take no notice of them.

  ii. A handy guide that can ring alarm bells on occasions.

  iii. Useful to read, if I have the time.

SPIRIT ASSESSMENT

16. If at first you don't succeed, try, try again. Is this true for you?

  i. Mostly true, but some days it can be more of an effort.

  ii. What's the point?

  iii. Absolutely true!

17. On average, in a week, how much quiet time do you put aside for yourself?

  i. It's just not on my radar.

  ii. If I'm lucky, 30 minutes or so.

  iii. I try to make it a regular consideration.

18. How do you feel you cope with stress?

  i. I know I can only change what I have control over.

  ii. Not well. Eating is one of my comfort blankets.

  iii. I believe in rowing my boat gently down the stream, not up!

THE MESSAGE IN THE MADNESS – THE MEANING BEHIND THE QUESTIONS

MIND ASSESSMENT

Question 1. What is your relationship with food?

Striking up a healthy and balanced relationship with food is a positive thing. To eat consciously and enjoy each mouthful is an art in itself, and the occasional overindulgence is fine too. Mainly, get to know your body so that you stop when you feel full.

Food fills a physical hunger but no amount of eating will fill an emotional hunger. If your emotional cravings are for positive feelings, dig deep as to how you can meet the root cause of the problem. Often, this comes down to feeling negative about yourself. Invest time and effort in the process of making friends with yourself. Treat yourself as you would like others to treat you. There's more on this on page 214.

  𝄞 Take pleasure in simple things

Question 2. What do you ask yourself when things aren't going your way?

If your quality of life lacks richness, start by exploring your inner questions, those you ask yourself. Questions direct your focus and determine your reality. The common question, 'Why can't I do "x"?', sends a message to your brain to start searching for all the reasons as to why you can't! It also assumes there is something to be done and that you are unable to do it. Conversely, you can train yourself to ask helpful and empowering questions like, 'What can I learn from this?' or 'How can I do this differently?' Your brain will continue to find a positive solution. In other words, the answer is only as helpful as the question.

Question 3. Think of a goal you have right now. How are you thinking about the goal?
How you think usually dictates the result. Your ability to think about what you really do want will increase the likelihood of achieving the goal. Those who think about what they don't want are likely to achieve just that. For example, if you tell yourself not to worry, you are instructing your brain to worry. If you are thinking of slimming, do you imagine yourself slim and energetic or are you thinking of the foods you must avoid and the amount of weight you have to lose? If you are thinking of being confident, that becomes much more likely. What you think influences how you feel and how you act. There's more on this on page 3.

🐾 *Do what you love and learn to love what you do*

BODY ASSESSMENT
Question 4. What's your waist measurement?
Trim waists are in, it's official. If you can't see your waist this signifies fat around your belly, which can be much more risky than fat around your hips. If you are overweight but most of the fat is lurking in your hips, then you're considered healthier than someone of the same weight with a high-risk waist measurement. Too much fat lying around on your tummy can mean there is a lot of fat lying around in your blood. This can make

you more prone to conditions such as insulin resistance (where your body doesn't respond well to its own insulin, a hormone), high blood cholesterol, type 2 diabetes and high blood pressure. So it may make sense to throw out the bathroom scales and make friends with a measuring tape instead.

Question 5. What is your BMI?
Body mass index, or BMI, is used internationally to assess whether you have a healthy weight or not. If you fall within the 20–24 range, then you're likely to have the lowest risk of ill-health. Remember though, that being less than this (underweight), can also be linked to health problems such as osteoporosis and lowered immunity. So don't be fooled into emulating the skinny models and celebrities in magazines. And if you find you're creeping into the 'overweight' or 'obese' category, you'll have to work a little harder. Take pride if you fall within the healthy BMI.

It's best to look at BMI as well as your waist measurement, rather than BMI in isolation. Indeed, here's a surprise. If you want even more of a body assessment, you could try measuring your body fat using body fat monitoring scales. Knowing that you're carrying more muscle and less fat can be a great boost to the ego.

❧ Live your own life, not someone else's

Question 6. Your body shape can best be described as …
Your body shape is partly inherited, so if you come from a pear-shaped family, you just got lucky. There's a wealth of research that shows that being apple-shaped (having a waist that's larger than your hips) appears to be associated with health risks. Although you may simply want to lose weight so that you look more stun-

ning, take a moment to think about how shedding those pounds may give you many more years of good health. A larger waist has been associated with higher blood cholesterol, which can make you more prone to heart disease, especially if you smoke or are inactive.

Being apple-shaped can also increase your risk of a condition called metabolic syndrome (also known as Syndrome X or insulin resistance) which can lead to type 2 diabetes. Balanced low-GI eating is a fantastic way of helping to prevent diabetes in people who already have metabolic syndrome. It's thought that this problem affects around one in five adults in the UK – and many don't even know it. So, eating the Hot Body way could make a significant difference to your health and you could be preventing problems you didn't even know you had!

❞❧ *There is no failure, only learning*

PHYSICAL ASSESSMENT

Question 7. How do you feel about physical activity?
Whatever you don't use, you lose. It's easy to see this in your physical body. If you stop using your legs they will stop working! Moving around and exercising is great news for your body and enhances the use of your brain, too. Incorporating regular activity helps to mobilise your fat stores, and burn calories, so you lose weight even more effectively.

Question 8. How much exercise do you get on average?
Whatever your age, the recommended daily dose of activity burst on our Hot Body Plan is two 10-minute sessions of moderately intense activity. Being active doesn't mean you have to do a planned 'exercise' in the form of a fitness class or gym. Getting

off your chair at home or work, and moving around can have an impact. When you make moving a habit, it will help you feel less lethargic. There's more on this in Chapter Six: Get GiP-fit.

Question 9. Which statement best applies to you, regarding physical activity?
Exercise is often linked with a healthy self-image and can become a positive addiction! The key is to choose an activity you enjoy and that fits in with your lifestyle. When you get it right, you're likely to find that it produces more and more pleasure and you begin to experience a new-found level of vitality and energy.

❧ Be conscious of your eating

FOOD ASSESSMENT
Question 10. How many colours are there on your plate, on average?
Think of a colourful fruit or vegetable bowl. Imagine the bright orange satsumas, yellow bananas, rich green Granny Smiths and Red Delicious apples, purple plums, green broccoli, red cabbage, purple beetroot, orange carrots and any other favourites you might have. This isn't just about vitamin C. Each different colour of fruit and vegetables can provide you with a different health benefit. For example, the orange colour in carrots gives you beta-carotene, which your body converts into vitamin A. You need vitamin A to keep your skin, eyes and immune system healthy. Similarly, the purple pigment in plums and blueberries contains anthocyanins, which are powerful antioxidants. And the potent lycopene in tomatoes, especially processed tomatoes, has been shown to have cancer-fighting properties. In short, eat a rainbow!

Question 11. Your meal and snack habits tend to be ...
Eating regularly can help to prevent hunger pangs. Missing meals can sometimes make you ravenous by your next meal or snack time and this could mean you reach for something quick, convenient and calorific. Instead, eat regular meals and light snacks, around five to six times a day. This also helps keep your blood sugar levels even and steady throughout the day, especially because this plan is based on low-GI eating. There's more on this on page 12.

Question 12. Alcohol is like ...
There is evidence to show that small amounts of alcohol may be beneficial to your heart. And it's the *small* that is the operative word! A glass of wine with your meal is fine. It's when you choose to go for half a bottle that the calories and undesirable effects mount up. Keep to the recommended limits, as shown on page 115.

❧ Adopt an easy, accepting and uncomplicated philosophy

Question 13. Which carb do you eat most often?
Different carbs have different effects on your blood sugar. Most types of pasta, especially if they are cooked al dente, will give you the nice slow, steady rise in blood glucose that helps you to keep to the Hot Body Plan. But remember, it isn't about piling on the pasta, as that could pile on the pounds too. Have controlled amounts as suggested in our carb boxes on pages 82–6.

Some types of rice, such as sticky rice, used in risottos, can make your blood glucose rise quickly, so it's best to go for slowly digested types such as basmati or brown rice. And it might surprise you to know that wholemeal bread makes your blood glucose rise just as quickly as white bread. This is because the wheat grains have been ground up, making them much quicker to digest. Remember, though, wholemeal bread does have more fibre and B vitamins, so it's not a bad food. Next time you're ordering your sandwich, consider whether seeded or granary bread might make a nice lower-GI change. Even white bread with seeds in it will be digested more slowly than wholemeal bread.

Question 14. Do you eat breakfast …
Okay, you've heard the 'eat like a prince in the morning and like a pauper in the evening' saying far too many times for it to register anything now. But, for a moment, just think about what happens in your body. If you take in more calories in the daytime, you're more likely to use them up as you're rushing around either at work, at home or even in the supermarket. This rushing-around helps you to use up some of the calories that you ate in the previous meal or snack. However, in the evening, particularly late in the evening, you're less likely to be active. So the calories you take in later on in the day are more likely to end up round your belly. Unless of course you change your routine and go for a walk round the block after your evening meal – possible?

Breakfast particularly helps you to break that overnight fast. As you sleep, your blood glucose level goes down and this means there is less sugar supplied to your brain. In the morning, when you need to be alert and able to perform, it's important to get that sugar to your brain and to keep it there for a few hours. A balanced low-GI breakfast will help you do just that.

Question 15. When you shop for food, are the labels …
Not many of us have the time to scrutinise the small print on a food label when at the supermarket. The Food Standards Agency has recognised this, as have many grocery chains and food manufacturers. You may have noticed new simpler labelling that is colour-coded for easy reference on some food packaging. Here's the low-down.

Stop at the red light!
New traffic light colour codes on pre-packaged foods have been introduced by the Food Standards Agency. They guide you on the amounts of fat, saturated fat, sugar and salt in 100 g of a particular food.

Green = *Low*
Amber = *Medium*
Red = *High*

To help you lose weight and also maintain good health, it's best to cut down on saturated fat, salt and added sugars, so choosing foods that are closer to green and amber in fat, salt and sugar will help you to make healthier choices. If you see a red light, stop and think. Does this food get me closer to the Hot Body I desire?

Since packaged foods are made up of lots of ingredients, you will find that the traffic light labels will have some greens, some ambers and some reds. If you're comparing two brands, go for the one that has more green and amber and, just like when you're driving, try to avoid too many red lights.

Some manufacturers have chosen to give information on Guideline Daily Amounts (GDAs) on the front of their packaging. GDAs are guidelines for healthy adults and children about the approximate amount of calories, fat, saturated fat, carbohydrate, total sugars, protein, fibre, salt and sodium required for a healthy diet.

Nutrient	GDAs for WOMEN
Energy (Calories)	2000
Fat (g)	70
Saturated fat (g)	20
Carbohydrate (g)	230
Total sugars (g)	90
Dietary fibre (AOAC) (g)	24
Dietary fibre (NSP) (g)	18
Sodium (g)	2.4
Salt (g)	6

It is very difficult – and indeed impractical – for you to achieve the GDAs for all nutrients in any one day. GDAs are there to act as a guide and to help you to compare products. In this way, you could compare the amount of fat per serving in two different brands of the same food.

✿ Wake up to a happy thought

SPIRIT ASSESSMENT
Question 16. If at first you don't succeed, try, try again. Is this true for you?

Events don't reveal a person – they make a person. If you do what you always do, you'll get what you've always got! Mental flexibility is the key here. Life's challenges can bring great growth, if you let them. Consider one of your goals. What are you doing now to achieve it? The more choices you open up to, the higher the chances of you succeeding. If one of your chosen options isn't working, choose another and another until you find the one.

Question 17. On average, in a week, how much quiet time do you put aside for yourself?
Building in 'me' moments is hugely beneficial in terms of nurturing and nourishing your soul. Practise becoming a human be-ing, as opposed to a human do-ing! Basically, give yourself permission to enjoy your own company, even if it's only for 15 minutes a day. Take a 'me' moment to see the new you with a spirit of joy and lightness around you. *Hear* the sounds of laughter or giggles coming from within you. Alternatively, hear the sound of silence and *feel* the surge of lightness and joy enveloping you. There's more on this on page 48.

De-clutter your mind by ridding yourself of unnecessary burdens such as possessions and, in some instances, even people. Simplify your life and your environments. When you nourish your mind and spirit, you will be mentally stronger in paying better attention to your physical needs. This includes the likelihood of healthier eating and taking regular exercise. A gradual weight loss means a sustainable result. If it's worth having, it's worth the gradual but lasting results! There's more on this on page 53.

❧ Get a good night's sleep

Question 18. How do you feel you cope with stress?
It is not always possible to have control over events that take place on the outside, but you always have control over how you interpret and respond to something in yourself. One way is to choose to perceive that everything in your life is not there by

coincidence and therefore for good reasons. Appreciate all you have and be thankful for what you don't have! Eliminate conflict by following the path of least resistance, surround yourself with joyful people and laugh a lot! There's more on this on page 220.

HOW DID YOU SCORE?

Key

1.	i) =	2	ii) =	1	iii) =	3
2.	i) =	1	ii) =	3	iii) =	2
3.	i) =	3	ii) =	1	iii) =	2
4.	i) =	2	ii) =	3	iii) =	1
5.	i) =	3	ii) =	2	iii) =	1
6.	i) =	1	ii) =	3	iii) =	2
7.	i) =	3	ii) =	1	iii) =	2
8.	i) =	2	ii) =	1	iii) =	3
9.	i) =	1	ii) =	2	iii) =	3
10.	i) =	2	ii) =	3	iii) =	1
11.	i) =	3	ii) =	2	iii) =	1
12.	i) =	1	ii) =	3	iii) =	2
13.	i) =	1	ii) =	3	iii) =	2
14.	i) =	3	ii) =	1	iii) =	2
15.	i) =	1	ii) =	3	iii) =	2
16.	i) =	2	ii) =	1	iii) =	3
17.	i) =	1	ii) =	2	iii) =	3
18.	i) =	2	ii) =	1	iii) =	3

41–54 points: you're at the **GREEN LIGHT**
29–40 points: you're at the **AMBER LIGHT**
18–28 points: you're at the **RED LIGHT**

WHAT DOES YOUR SCORE SAY ABOUT YOU?

GREEN LIGHT

Pukka job done, gold star, Queen of the dance floor. There's nothing stopping you now, carry on making the fantastic choices you make and you could be oozing with even more confidence. Continuing on this green path, and following the handy tips in this book, will mean that you're more likely to maintain a healthy body weight, forever.

AMBER LIGHT

Well done for getting closer to your goal. Now's your chance to build on the changes that you've made and propel yourself towards greener choices. Eating regularly, moving around more and making sure you have nourishing low-GI choices at every meal will ensure you are well on your way to fitting into that little black number. Make a decision now to take on three simple weight-loss tips from this book, and watch how this makes a difference to your waistline and your wow! factor. As you begin to see results, take on another couple of tips or try a new recipe and gradually carry on, slowly and surely. Remember that even losing one or two pounds is making a difference.

RED LIGHT

Okay, time to stop and think. You picked up this book for a reason. There is something in you that has made you decide to get on and fulfil that dream of being slimmer, healthier, more confident, and so on. It's time to evaluate what's important to you in your life. Losing just 5 per cent of your weight has myriad health effects – reduces the strain on your back and knees, reduces breathlessness, reduces your risk of developing cancer, heart disease and more, lifts your mood and self-esteem and even improves your sex life. What would happen if you started today?

AND FINALLY...

✳ Use relaxation tapes regularly. When you are stressed, your body releases certain hormones to help you combat that stress. What you may not realise is that the same hormones can also raise your blood sugar. Lower your stress levels and you're more likely to have steady blood sugar levels.

✳ Research shows that people who eat breakfast find it easier to lose weight.

✳ Chew your food slowly and savour every mouthful. This can help you to feel more satisfied, discouraging overeating.

✳ Get into the habit of finishing dinner around four hours before you go to bed. This helps you to have some time to digest the meal and to use up those calories before you go to sleep.

✳ Most people will finish what's on their plate or what's in the pack. Use smaller plates and buy smaller packs and you'll curb overindulgence.

CHAPTER THREE: HOW HOT BODIED IS YOUR LIFE?

Try our quiz and get a snap shot of where you are by answering the questions honestly.

QUIZ: TEST YOUR REACTIONS

1. *When you can no longer fit into your favourite jeans, what are you most likely to do?*
a) Adopt a more confident posture by standing straighter and sucking in the stomach muscles.
b) Think about building in more physical activity and re-evaluating your diet, but do very little about it!
c) Use it as a good excuse for a new wardrobe.

2. *When you 'go on a diet', what are you likely to do?*
a) Eat less.
b) Cut out carbs, fats or sweets.
c) Embrace the latest 'in' celeb diet.

3. *What's your relationship with alcohol?*
a) Don't drink / social drinker.
b) Occasionally binge.
c) A daily drink is a must!

4. *If you experience a drop in energy levels, what do you do?*

a) Get outdoors and go for a walk.

b) Grab some sneaky shut-eye.

c) Head for the coffee or snack machine.

5. *When you really feel short of hours in a day, which of these is likely to be sacrificed?*

a) TV and DVDs.

b) Meeting up with mates.

c) A meal or exercise.

6. *Which one of these most applies to you when you feel under stress?*

a) Practise breathing deeply.

b) Take it out on others.

c) Nose bag!

7. *How do you manage in your own company?*

a) You're chilled. You enjoy time on your own.

b) You're uncomfortable but you manage.

c) You feel anxious and look to find someone to call or meet up with.

8. *With a bonus of some spare minutes, how do you choose to spend them?*

a) Enjoy the peace and calm of the moment.

b) Phone a friend or watch TV.

c) Snack attack!

9. *When you are unhappy in a partnership or are experiencing confrontational or difficult relationships, how do you react?*

a) Put yourself in their shoes to work on possible solutions and share your feelings in a clear-headed way.

b) Avoid further confrontation/get out fast.
c) Get defensive or blame yourself, for a long while afterwards.

10. When you feel upset by someone, how do you handle the emotions?

a) Acknowledge the feelings and whether the remark/action was intended in 'that' way.
b) Confront the person.
c) Hurt them back or suffer in silence.

HOW DID YOU SCORE?

MAINLY A)

You know the importance of remaining on an even keel and nurturing balance in all areas of your life. Whatever your indulgences, you recognise choices and consequences. When in doubt, press your imaginary pause button to consider an emotionally intelligent response.

MAINLY B)

You may find yourself constantly making adjustments so as not to fall into unhealthy habits. And, all credit to you for doing so. Your actions will speak louder than words, so consider each of your responses and whether your choice in that moment is taking you nearer to what you ultimately want.

MAINLY C)

When the pain outweighs the pleasure, you may choose to make the changes and/or get the support that will enable you to feel great about yourself. Focusing on what you really want will help you to stay on track as you naturally gravitate towards your dominant thoughts, followed by your actions.

❧ *Develop your mental and physical flexibility*

IS YOUR MIND ON YOUR SIDE?

Hopefully, this little exercise has helped you see a little better where you are in your life and what you want to achieve. Maybe you already know that you're 'up for it' and just want to get on and shed a few inches or pounds. Perhaps you just want to appreciate your body and quite simply, feel sexier, more appealing and happier. If so, there are a few tips below that can get you started, then skip the last section (from 'Work from the Inside, Out') and go straight to Chapter Four: The GiP Factor – and get going.

But maybe you have other issues that need to be tackled first. Perhaps life's signposts are out, telling you that the imbalances that you are experiencing need addressing. Maybe your relationship has lost its get up and go. If so, see below – 'Work from the Inside, Out' until you feel ready to really tackle the Hot Body Plan.

TIP ONE: *Keep fit – it's so de-stressing!*
Negotiating the maze of busyness, whether it's being a taxi service for the kids, talking and ironing simultaneously or shovelling your meal down with seconds to spare, en route to the next 'must be seen at' event, no wonder you feel stressed! Experts cannot emphasise enough the importance of building in regular physical activity in order to manage and significantly reduce stress levels.

So, if you recognise yourself as being a 'busy – talk to me when I have more time!' type, get to scheduling in your fitness. Other priorities can easily get in the way, so write it down and commit to it. There's something about writing it down that makes owning it more powerful. Find a supportive buddy and agree your timings, preferably a week in advance.

> 🐾 'Finding someone who inspires you, a role model or even just a friend or partner who gently encourages you with any goal can be of huge benefit. My hubby recently changed jobs. One of his conscious outcomes was to work locally and find a place of work with a gym attached! So guess what? Yep! That's what he found, in a role that he enjoys! This conscious creation means he cycles to work and back, a round trip of around one and a half hours, then works out in the gym before he starts his working day. He gets the bus in on Fridays so as he can rest his legs ready for league hockey every Saturday! And on Sundays, the day of rest (!), we either cycle along the coast with the dog playing catch up, or take a gentle stroll over the Downs.'

In addition to the many great reasons for daily physical activity, add to them a more youthful face! As your heart pumps blood around, you become flushed with colour and as you sweat, you lessen any swelling in your face, too. Exercise releases those feel-good chemicals and leaves you feeling upbeat, relaxed and more motivated and determined to achieve your goals. After even a 10-minute workout, you are likely to notice those warm glowing cheeks.

TIP TWO: *Water it down*

So, you want to be in with the 'in crowd'? Join the celebs, and never be seen without it – water, that is! Here's how drinking plenty of water can help you:

✻ Acts as a natural appetite suppressant
✻ Reduces bloating
✻ Gives radiant skin
✻ Aids sound sleep
✻ Reduces headaches
✻ Helps kidney function
✻ And possibly more!

Often when you think you are hungry, you are actually thirsty. So, try drinking water when you feel hungry. This could be all you need and you might save yourself shovelling in extra calories – all helping you to manage your weight.

Less bloating around the abdomen means a flatter stomach and noticeably better-fitting clothes. Around eight to ten glasses a day should do it and you can start off with less, just gradually build up – add a slice of lemon or drink it hot as mint tea if you fancy a change. It's so easily available that you forget what this miracle product offers. The best functional food in the universe!

❧ Eat little and often

TIP THREE: *Eat chocolate!*

Yes, it's true! A little of what you fancy does do you good. When you are fixated about going on a diet, what you think about expands! So, you focus more on all the naughty but nice foods that you shouldn't, mustn't, can't have and food depriva-tion encourages the brain to choose the easiest path of least resistance, meaning, ditch the diet! In this way, you are inadvertently sabotaging the goal that you really want, which may be to fit into your much loved little black number or favourite pair of jeans.

With the Hot Body Plan, you can allow yourself a regular treat, be it a glass of wine or a small choc bar, over the next 28 days. If your body was a classic car, you would fill it with the best petrol to ensure it runs smoothly. Treat your body in the same way and remember that when the tank is full, stop filling it!

Now, if you feel you are ready, turn to the next chapter – The GiP Factor – and get started on building the new 'you'. If you feel you still need a little more motivation, read on ...

WORK FROM THE INSIDE, OUT

You'd be surprised at how many attractive women, models too, have hang-ups about their body image and are convinced that they are fat and unattractive! The downward spiral is the more unattractive you feel, the more this shows in your behaviour and actions, from the inside, out. If you currently cringe when you look in the mirror, it will be challenging to present yourself 'out there', confidently.

In the fast and furious times that we live in, it can, on occasion, be easy to lose the plot! Prevention is better than cure, and balance, in all aspects of your life, helps you to remain on an even keel. If you don't make time to look after your health, you are, in a sense, making time to get ill. Ill health comes from being out of kilter. Good health returns when you pay attention to your mental, physical and spiritual wellbeing. After all, you are the most important product of your life.

Be prepared to face any difficult feelings and take small bite-size steps to overcome and manage them. Seek support through a friend, GP or reputable counsellor. Food can only fill a physical hole but is no help when it comes to an emotional void. And, if you are prone to comfort eating, take the time out to work through your unmet need(s). Rather than trying to fill it with food, confront the suppressed emotion.

Changing your mental attitude to support a healthier lifestyle will enable you to enjoy your physical attributes as a result of this mental transformation. This is about rediscovering your inner beauty, power and acceptance of who you are, which often leads to the magical physical things that can happen as a result. Follow the guidance offered and delight in passing your reflection! So, what could you say to yourself on the inside that will engender a more attractive, confident outside?

❧ *Laugh a lot!*

ME, ME, ME, ME, ME!

You are the most important product of your life, so look after yourself. A simple truth is that without precious chill time, your awake time becomes less and less effective as you continue to chase your tail or someone else's! And, life is something that happens while you are making other plans.

How many of the following do you currently identify with?

✳ Never enough hours in a day
✳ Living in stress city
✳ Ineffective
✳ Tired and emotional!

One important realisation is that life goes on without you for that 30 minutes or so of time out. A tough one to get your head round, but true! Once you discover this and take a leap of faith by turning off the mobile, shutting the door, switching on the answerphone and whatever else, you are on your way to a more productive life. Choose any which way to use this time spent alone. Chances are, that the half hour out will increase your effectiveness in other areas, twofold, due to your increased energy, clearer mind and increased focus. This investment is one of the most important that you can make. You'll wonder how you did without it for so long. Let go of the martyr complex, if you know you are that way inclined, and enlist the support of others if you need to, especially if it means taking the kids off your hands.

&* *Watch funny DVDs*

YOUR X FACTOR

There are some amazing models of inspiration, and finding your shining star can help to drive you towards your own goals of success.

Consider and write down your answers to the following:

* Who inspires you?
* How would the new you look, sound and feel?
* What are your dreams and desires?

By *acting* as if you have already succeeded in accomplishing your goals, you are pretty much halfway there. Your mind doesn't easily recognise what's real and what's imagined. See yourself with a brighter smile, a twinkle in your eyes, an upright posture, and oozing with self-confidence. Put up a photo of your role model (it could even be a past picture of you), somewhere you are likely to see it frequently. You can change it every so often, too. This will help you to maintain a high level of motivation.

Feeling great on the inside shows on the outside in many ways, including your behaviour, and will support you in developing the qualities and capabilities that you desire most. It's a whole package that links together. Increasing your self-confidence can impact on many other areas of your life: going for the job you really want or even changing career direction, for example.

LET IT OUT!

Breathing is good and breathing consciously is even better! Especially if you want to improve these areas:

✳ Managing anxiety or stress
✳ Managing fear (False Evidence Appearing Real!)
✳ Trusting your feelings and choices
✳ Increasing your focus

Breathing deeply and slowly enhances the effectiveness of your organs and circulatory system. On the other hand, shallow breathing can have a negative effect on your physical being, and can bring on feelings of anxiety. As with conscious eating, conscious deep breathing can help you to tap into your emotions and deeper feelings.

The secret to achieving this, is to simply place your hand on your belly so that when you inhale, your belly expands as you push it out and contracts as you exhale.

🐦 *Simplify your life*

VISUALISATION EXERCISE

Try this: in your imagination, pick a place where you can experience a wonderful sense of calm and relaxation. It could be anywhere, like a beach, woods or mountains. Now use your senses to 'be there' for real. See the scenery in detail and make the images bright and colourful. What are you hearing? Pay attention to the laughter, silence, birds singing, waves lapping over the rocks, or anything else. What can you feel? Perhaps it's the warmth of the sun, or the freshness of the mountain air or even the wind brushing against your face. Pay attention to your feelings – and enjoy the peace and serenity for a few more minutes. Practise your deep breathing as you do so.

Laughing is another highly enjoyable way to chill and loosen you up. When chaos reigns and your world feels like it's seen better days, laughter can quite literally be the best medicine, ever! As you shake off those tensions, releasing the anxieties, your breathing becomes more efficient. Have something in reserve for those times when you most need cheering up. This could be a funny person in your life that you are blessed with, watching the antics of an animal or child, or a funny film that you know will make you howl.

AND FINALLY...

✷ Physical activity is a great combination for reducing stress and mentally clearing your mind while burning the calories and nourishing your spirit.

✷ When you feel hungry, it could actually be your body telling you you're thirsty. Drink a glass of water and move on.

✳ Know what you want, write it down and read and repeat it several times in the day, especially when you wake in the mornings and just before you fall asleep.

✳ Convince your mind that you already have succeeded in reaching your goal, visualising what you see, hear and feel.

✳ Be aware of opportunities that will help you and those that will not. Remain focused and energised. You have the power and the discipline if you want it enough.

CHAPTER FOUR:
THE GiP FACTOR

Many diets promote rapid weight loss with tag lines such as 'Lose a stone in two weeks'. We're not into quick fixes. We don't believe this is healthy or sustainable and therefore we recommend you lose around ½–1 kg (1–2 lb) each week. In just 28 days, you could lose around 3 kg – half a stone – which is steady and sensible and, more importantly, sustainable in the long term. The Hot Body Plan is full of flavour and flexibility. It's like going into a sweet shop and picking and mixing your favourite combinations to savour, only this time it's not going to show on your waistline. This plan is based on eating foods that fill you up, are slowly digested and help you to lose weight slowly and steadily.

Our weight-loss plan is based on incorporating healthy low-GI foods into your everyday meals and snacks. A simple way to do this is to eat more high-fibre foods, such as a wholegrain cereal or muesli for breakfast; balanced lower-fat meals with low-GI carbs (such as pasta or multigrain bread) and vegetables/salad on the side; and tasty snacks in between.

Choose foods that need more chewing

THE GIP FACTOR

Calculating GI or calories can be boring and impractical. That's why we've devised our unique GiP system that's done all the calculating for you. You don't need to do any counting, just pick 'n' mix the food choices, as shown below. Since everyone is different everyone will lose weight at different rates. However, on average, you should find that the choices in this plan will help you lose the recommended ½–1 kg (1–2 lb) per week or around 3 kg (7 lb) in 28 days.

If you're losing weight too quickly, simply allow yourself some more low-GI carbs each day (such as a slice of soya and linseed bread, or a banana). Conversely, if you're not losing this amount per week, cut back a little on your portion sizes and be very aware of your cooking methods so that you're keeping your fat intake down.

WHAT YOU DO

✳ Choose a breakfast.

✳ Choose two main meals by following the guidelines below. Include a piece of fruit for dessert, or if you are struggling with all the veggies, substitute one portion of veg for a piece of fruit.

✳ Choose two snacks in between meals.

✳ Use 200 ml (7 fl oz) semi-skimmed (or skimmed) milk each day for drinks throughout the day.

✳ Use low-fat spread very sparingly, that is, no more than 1 teaspoon on a slice of bread. If you use butter, make it half a teaspoon.

✳ Add a teaspoon of olive oil or rapeseed oil in cooking for the day if you want to. You can also use a few sprays of spray oil in cooking.

✳ Enjoy the free drinks and flavourings as shown.

✳ Have a maximum of seven units of alcohol a week – but try to have a few alcohol-free days each week (see page 115). Remember that alcohol lowers your blood sugar levels and so may leave you feeling hungry.

YOUR DAILY CHECKLIST

Breakfast	1 from list
Free veggies	4 servings
Protein portions	2 servings
Carb portions	2 servings
Fruit	2 servings, 1 as part of each main meal (or have diet yoghurt as a dessert)
Snacks	2, at least 1 being fruit
Milk, semi- or skimmed	200 ml (7 fl oz) for beverages
Dairy foods	Make sure that as well as your milk above you include two lower-fat dairy based foods from the protein portions (e.g. lower-fat cheese), breakfasts (e.g. semi-skimmed milk) or snacks (e.g. diet yoghurt)
Water, tea, coffee, low-calorie squash, low-calorie flavoured waters	6–8 cups or glasses a day
And get physical!	Two 10-minute bursts of moderately intense activity

BE PREPARED

You are embarking on a new lifestyle. It's easy and fun, but it will only be so if you have the recommended foods accessible – and don't have the unhealthy but possibly tempting foods sitting in front of you, ready to sabotage your goals.

Read through this chapter and make a list of the sort of foods you would like to eat for the next few days. Consider if it's better to take some snacks to work; what sort of veggies you like, so you have plenty for your main meals; free flavourings you may need for cooking to help you trim the fat and turn up the taste, any ingredients for recipes you fancy, and so on. Here are some basic prep tips to help you ease into your new lifestyle smartly and effortlessly:

✳ Buy chicken breasts, cut into strips and freeze in small freezer bags. You can then quickly defrost them and use them for a speedy stir-fry or some chicken fajitas. You could even cook them in advance and freeze them, so you have cooked chicken all set for sandwiches.

✳ Boil a large pot of pasta and freeze it in small containers for the freezer. This could come in really handy when you want to have a quick pasta dish: just stir in some tomato-based pasta sauce and throw in a can of beans or sweetcorn – delicious, quick and healthy. Add a huge salad for extra balance.

✳ Have lots of raw veggies in the fridge so you can make carrot sticks, veg crudités or a snack attack box (see page 103). You can have any of these with a clear conscience as they are low-GI, low in calories and high in crunch. You'll find they're a lifesaver for taking to work or for in-between meal munchies or for digging into when you come home hungry and need a quick fix.

* Give away your party leftovers, and any unhealthy snacks you have lurking in the larder. Out of sight really can be out of mind.

* Invest in some time-savers and calorie-cutters: non-stick pans, spray bottle for your favourite cooking oil, sandwich toaster, healthy grill, and so on.

TO START OFF YOUR SHOPPING LIST ...

Diet hot chocolate powder

Fat-free dressings – choose two or three different types for variety

Lower-fat tomato-based pasta sauces (compare labels and choose lower-fat option)

Any variety of dried or fresh pasta, different shapes, as desired

Canned beans and lentils, such as kidney beans, chickpeas and pinto beans

Olive or rapeseed spray oil

Roasted peanuts in shells or small packets of peanuts (ideally unsalted), almonds and/or walnuts

Salad vegetables

Frozen vegetables

Fresh fruit

Dried fruit

Granary, seeded or lower-GI breads

Pitta bread or wraps

Coarse grain or regular mustard

New potatoes

Oatcakes

> Diet yoghurt
>
> Low-fat natural yoghurt
>
> Other lower-fat dairy products, such as semi- or skimmed milk, ricotta cheese
>
> Easy cook or basmati rice

THE PLAN

Here are your meal ideas. Note that we mention some brands and some retailers. This doesn't mean to say we think these are the best brands or that we recommend you use these retailers. It's just that we only have GI data from these common foods, so we can't give you information on foods from other manufacturers and retailers at this time. However this Hot Body Plan, as you know, is about using your common sense, so if you see a food that seems very similar to one listed here (such as a different brand of raw porridge oats), then go for it. Your weight loss and fullness factor will tell you whether you're on the right track.

    🖎 *Try our 15-minute tasty recipes*

1. CHOOSE YOUR BREAKFAST

Here are some winning combinations of low-GI (slowly digested) breakfast ideas.

CEREAL DAY

5 tbsp All Bran and up to 200 ml (7 fl oz) skimmed or semi-skimmed milk

* * *

2 wheat biscuits and up to 200 ml (7 fl oz) skimmed or semi-skimmed milk

* * *

3–4 tbsp muesli with 150 ml (5 fl oz) skimmed or semi-skimmed milk

* * *

Half a bowl (25 g/1 oz) Tesco High Fibre Bran and up to 200 ml (7 fl oz) skimmed or semi-skimmed milk

* * *

8 tbsp made-up porridge (regular, rolled oats are better than instant) made with water as per pack instructions. Add 1 tbsp dried fruit or 1 tsp sugar or honey if you like.

* * *

6 tbsp made-up porridge (regular is better than instant) made with 100 ml (4 fl oz) skimmed or semi-skimmed milk and water as required. Add 1 tbsp dried fruit or 1 tsp sugar or honey if you like.

* * *

3 tbsp (40 g/1½ oz) raw Sainsbury's Taste the Difference Scottish Jumbo Oats cooked in 150 ml (5 fl oz) skimmed or semi-skimmed milk. Add 1 tbsp dried fruit or 1 tsp sugar or honey if you like.

* * *

Half a bowl (40 g/1½ oz) Sainsbury's Whole Grain Mini-wheats and 150–200 ml (5–7 fl oz) skimmed or semi-skimmed milk

* * *

3 tbsp (40 g/1½ oz) Tesco Value Muesli and up to 200 ml (7 fl oz) skimmed or semi-skimmed milk

* * *

5 tbsp Sainsbury's Puffed Wheat and up to 200 ml (7 fl oz) skimmed or semi-skimmed milk

* * *

2 Weetabix and up to 200 ml (7 fl oz) skimmed or semi-skimmed milk

5 tbsp Sainsbury's Puffed Wheat with sliced strawberries and up to 200 ml (7 fl oz) skimmed or semi-skimmed milk. Add an artificial sweetener if you like.

* * *

4 tbsp bran flakes with up to 200 ml (7 fl oz) skimmed or semi-skimmed milk
Glass of tomato juice with a dash of Worcestershire sauce

BREADY DAY

Small glass of unsweetened fruit juice (150 ml/5 fl oz)
1 slice multigrain bread, toasted, with a scraping of half-fat, unsaturated or low-fat spread or butter and 1 level tsp reduced-sugar jam

* * *

2 tsp peanut butter and half a sliced banana on 1 slice seeded bread or toast. No more nuts allowed today if you choose this.

* * *

2 boiled eggs
Fresh or canned tomatoes, if desired
1 slice granary toast or M & S Oatmeal Soft Farmhouse toast with a scraping of half-fat, unsaturated or low-fat spread

* * *

Wholegrain bread (2 slices) or one M & S Two in One Muffin with 3 tsp Nutella hazelnut spread
Small glass of fruit juice

* * *

2 tsp peanut butter on 1 slice seeded bread or toast, scraping of reduced-sugar jam (optional). No more nuts allowed today if you choose this.

* * *

2 slices M & S Two in One Bread with low-fat spread

1 boiled egg

* * *

2 slices pumpernickel bread with scraping of butter, 1 tsp marmalade
1 small glass of orange juice

FRUITY DAY

Almond and strawberry yoghurt:
Mix together 2 tbsp chopped almonds and a strawberry diet yoghurt. No more nuts allowed today if you choose this.

* * *

Banana and melon pick-me-up:
1 under-ripe banana, sliced, mixed with half a cantaloupe melon, chopped. Serve chilled. Add a few strawberries if in season.

* * *

2 thin slices toasted raisin bread topped with sautéed mushrooms (sliced mushrooms sautéed in 10 sprays of oil and dried herbs)

* * *

Nuts and raisins. Mix 2 tbsp of your favourite nuts with 1 tbsp sultanas or raisins. No more nuts allowed today if you choose this.

* * *

1 small banana and 4 dried dates

* * *

M & S Eat Well Fresh Fruit in a Bottle – Apple and Kiwi
2 fruits of your choice, such as satsumas, plums or pears

HUNGRY DAY

Smoked salmon with avocado and soft cheese:
Mix 3 slices of smoked salmon, chopped, with 100 g (4 oz) ricotta cheese, season and pile into half an avocado. Scatter with 1 tsp of sesame seeds and serve with firm cherry tomatoes and lemon wedges

Cooked breakfast:
I poached egg, I rasher grilled lean bacon, grilled mushrooms
or mushrooms sautéed in 5 sprays of spray oil, chargrilled tomatoes or canned tomatoes
I slice multigrain toast

* * *

Vegetarian cooked breakfast:
I poached egg, half a small can of baked beans in tomato sauce,
grilled mushrooms or mushrooms sautéed in 5 sprays of spray
oil, chargrilled tomatoes or canned tomatoes
I slice multigrain toast

* * *

I scrambled egg (made with a little milk, seasoning, and scram-
bled in about ½ tsp of olive oil)
I slice multigrain bread, toasted
Grilled tomato halves, optional
Tesco Probiotic Orange or Cranberry Drink (Low GI)

* * *

2 poached eggs
Freshly grilled canned tomatoes flavoured with Worcestershire
sauce
I slice granary or wholegrain toast with a scraping of half-fat,
unsaturated or low-fat spread or yeast extract (e.g. Marmite)

* * *

2 slices Burgen Soya and Linseed Bread with a little low-fat spread
and I slice reduced-fat Edam cheese or 3 tbsp grated Cheddar

2. CHOOSE YOUR LUNCH OR DINNER: THE PICTURE YOUR PLATE PHILOSOPHY

This is the unique part of the Hot Body Plan. In this book, we've
made the GiP System even simpler. Imagine you have a couple

of chopsticks and you placed them across each other on top of your plate so that the plate is split into quarters. Two parts are to be filled with the veggies and/or salad (we call this the Veggie Veggie part), one with the meat, fish, pulses, egg or cheese (these are your Protein foods) and the last quarter is for the starchy food like potatoes, pasta or rice (the Carbs) – V V P C.

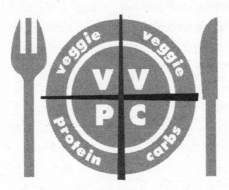

If you keep to this Hot Body V V P C (**V**eggie **V**eggie **P**rotein **C**arbs) plate model, you will instinctively be keeping to healthier proportions. Try thinking of meals as two veg plus meat, rather than meat and two veg. The vegetables are best treated as the main part of the meal. Having your plate piled up with veg and salad is a great way to make sure you get a range of vitamins and minerals. And they help to slow down the rate of digestion of the other foods on your plate, which in turn lowers the overall GI, helping you to feel fuller for longer.

❧ Have three calcium-rich foods a day

Now for the easy and flexible bit. Below you will see a range of boxes with the appropriate V V P C headings. Here are your guidelines:

✳ Pick one, two or even three choices from the veggie section, to fill the V V section of your plate.

✳ Choose one from the protein section – for example, a sandwich filling, a beanie salad or a piece of chicken or fish. Now three-quarters of your plate will be filled with food.

✳ Lastly select a carb from the carb boxes – bread if it's a sandwich; pasta or another choice if it's a plated meal.

✳ If you still want more after your meal, choose a fruit, unsweetened fruit juice or diet yoghurt. Whole fruit has plenty of fibre, so choose it more often than fruit juice. Having fruit after your meal is especially important if you have not quite managed to fill half your plate with veggies as it will help to lower the GI of your meal and keep you fuller for longer.

✳ If you fancy dabbling in the kitchen with one of our quick and easy recipes, then just follow the guidelines next to the recipe titles so you are still keeping in balance – taste not waist.

✳ Enjoy water, tea, coffee, unsweetened squash, diet drinks and sugar-free sparkling water. Use milk from your daily allowance of 200 ml (7 fl oz) semi-skimmed milk each day (skimmed if you prefer).

THE VEGGIE PART

✳ If you are opting for canned vegetables, then choose those canned in unsalted, unsweetened water (canned beans and sweetcorn kernels come under protein and carbs – there's more on this below).

✳ Fill up on veggies – remember to cover half of your plate and have more in between meals (as raw crudités, for example).

✳ Try to have at least two different veggies on your plate to give your meal colour and a variety of tastes and textures. Keep your meals interesting!

✳ Use a spray oil for cooking veg – they provide about 1 calorie per spray so even 10 sprays are no big deal.

✳ If you can't manage two veggies, then you can have some fruit (we talk about fruit later in this chapter). Better still is to have the two veggies and a portion of fruit!

Free Veggies – have as much as you like

Asparagus

Aubergines, grilled

Bamboo shoots

Bean sprouts

Beetroot

Broccoli

Brussels sprouts

Cabbage, white, green or red

Carrot, raw or steamed

Cauliflower

Celeriac

Celery

Chicory

Courgette, cooked in spray oil

Courgette, raw

Courgette, steamed

Cucumber, raw

Gherkins, pickled, drained

Green leafy veggies, e.g. spinach, curly kale

Leeks, steamed

Mange tout

Marrow

Mushrooms, grilled

Okra

Onions

Peppers, all colours

Pumpkin

Radish, red, raw

Runner beans

Salad leaves, any variety including lettuce

Spring onions

Swede, boiled

Sweetcorn, whole baby

Tomatoes, canned, with juice

Tomatoes, raw

Turnip, steamed or baked

Watercress

Other Veggies – have in the amounts shown

Baked beans, canned in tomato sauce	200 g (7 oz)	1 small can or ½ large can
Peas	75 g (3 oz)	3 level serving spoons
Sweetcorn kernels	75 g (3 oz)	2 rounded serving spoons

Veggie recipes

❧ Eat a rainbow of fruit and vegetables

10 things to do with vegetables

✳ Stuff large flat mushrooms with grated cheese and sun-dried tomatoes, and grill till the cheese has melted (this gives you one veg and one protein).

✳ Mix diced courgettes with crushed garlic and seasoning. Spray with one-calorie spray oil and microwave or stir-fry for 2–3 minutes.

✳ Make a salad with chopped tomatoes, lemon juice, oregano and coarse black pepper.

✳ Halve a courgette lengthways. Flavour with black pepper, ground cumin or curry powder. Add a little salt and some lemon juice. Microwave until just cooked – about a couple of minutes.

✳ Stir-fry a pack of quick stir-fry vegetables and flavour with chilli sauce and seasoning. Place the veggies in the centre of a tortilla wrap, top with crunchy cucumber and grated carrots and roll it into a Mexican veg fajita. All you need to add is protein – try 25 g (1 oz) grated Cheddar, or a generous serving of yoghurt-based garlic sauce or raita (for recipes, see pages 170–1).

∗ Scoop out the inside of a large tomato and fill it with a mixture of cottage cheese, chopped red apple and seasoning. This gives you one protein and one veg.

∗ Make a bean and pasta soup by mixing together tomato juice(v), your favourite canned beans(p), vegetable stock, dried thyme, chopped spring onion and cooked mini pasta shapes(c). All you need to add for a main meal is an after-dinner fruit as your extra veggie quarter.

∗ Cook French beans in a mixture of soy sauce and fresh or dried basil – just pop them into a greased microwavable dish and cook for a few minutes till tender. Sprinkle with some sesame seeds.

∗ Make a Thai salad with cucumber strips, bean sprouts, peppers, deseeded red chilli, coriander leaves, lime juice and a few drops of Thai fish sauce.

∗ Whip up a bean salad using any canned beans or sweet-corn, chopped celery, chopped tomatoes and red onions. Toss this in a fat-free dressing made from balsamic vinegar, a dash of honey and 1 tsp coarse grain mustard.

Can't find it?

If your favourite veggie doesn't appear on this list, it may be under starchy vegetables below (in which case it's counted under carbs, the C section of your plate), or we may not know its GI value and thus are unable to give it a GiP rating. Generally, most veggies are great and filling up on them instead of fatty foods makes sense.

Can't manage all that veg?

You will often see fruit and vegetables talked about together when you read an article on healthy eating. This is because they all generally contain a wide range of important nutrients for health. The richest sources of vitamins and minerals are fruit and vegetables. Vitamins and minerals are essential to health and play an important role in unleashing the energy stored in the other foods we eat and maintaining the fluid balance in tissue, and they are required for our muscles to function, all helping to maximise your workout! In addition to this, vital body functions, such as the immune system, are dependent on vitamins and minerals to work optimally.

So by choosing veggies interchangeably, as in the *five a day* message, you are still going to get lots of benefits. Sometimes you can't manage or just don't want to have half your plate filled with vegetables or salad. Since fruits offer similar ranges of nutrients, you can choose to have a fruit dessert but mentally 'count' it as though it were filling a quarter of your plate. There is more on this under the fruit section below.

HOW BIG IS YOUR PORTION?

While we have been talking about veggies we have been giving out a 'more the merrier' message, but that needs to change now that we come to the protein and carb parts of the Hot Body Plan. These foods will provide most of the energy (kcals or calories) in your diet, and of course to lose weight your energy/calorie intake needs to fall. All the scientific experiments on weight loss have shown that the more effective ways always include being very careful about portion sizes. It's easy to assume that a little extra of healthy foods can't be doing any harm, but beware! In my practice as a dietitian I see so many people who have a really healthy diet but are unable to lose weight because they are just eating too much of it.

The good news is that we have done the difficult part of portion control for you. On the following pages you will find that we have given recommended portion sizes for all the protein and carb foods. For each food we have given you a weight and a handy household or visual measure.

Why weigh?

You don't need to weigh any of your foods. Gauge your portion sizes the way you want to. Some people like the techie approach and prefer to weigh their food and it may be good for you to do this on the first occasion or two, just so you know what a portion size should look like. We have weights here for scientific completeness and it does avoid confusion where you may have similar foods in different sized packets.

Can't weigh, won't weigh…?

If you're about to give up before you start because the thought of scales leaves you cold, or they are just plain broken, then read on! The household and visual measures are there just for you. Why make life more difficult than it need be? Make the most of our background research – we have given the weights/measures to you, as keeping to the right portion sizes will be vital to your success. Of course, as you settle into your new exciting eating habits, these portions will become second nature and you will not need our help!

&. *Eat on a smaller plate*

Call a spoon a spoon?

A little research now on the spoons, cups and glasses in your kitchen will save time when planning and dishing up your meals. We suggest you get a few things out of your cupboards and spend a few minutes comparing your utensils to the standard ones we have used here in the book. A measuring jug with millilitre (ml) or fluid ounce (fl oz) markings or a set of kitchen measuring spoons will make this easier. Both are readily available in kitchenware shops or perhaps a friend can lend you some!

What we call it	Metric measurement	Imperial measurement
Teaspoon (tsp)	5 ml	n/a
Dessertspoon	10 ml	n/a
Tablespoon (tbsp)	15 ml	½ fl oz
Serving spoon	45 ml	1½ fl oz
Teacup or glass	200 ml	7 fl oz

If you don't have any teacups, then you may have a glass that will substitute as they usually have a 200 ml (7 fl oz) capacity, too.

For a guide on the size of measuring spoons and a 200ml glass, see page 238.

Also, note that unless otherwise stated:

✳ all spoons are level

✳ 3 tbsp = 1 serving spoon

THE PROTEIN PART

✳ Eggs – it's okay to have up to six per week, unless you have been advised to have less for a medical condition.

* Choose fish twice a week, one choice being oily fish, which is rich in heart-healthy omega-3 fats.

* Some dishes, such as beef stew, have been included because these foods have been tested for their GI rating. However, limit or avoid fat in cooking to keep the calories down.

* Poultry is a good choice, but note that the leg and thigh pieces can be high in saturated fat – chicken or turkey drumsticks with the skin on can have as many calories as fatty red meat! So, avoid the skin and choose breast cuts more often.

* You get three times as much if you use wafer-thin turkey or ham compared to standard thicker slices.

* Watch the salt – smoked foods or highly salted foods can make some people more prone to high blood pressure.

* The GI rating of turkey rashers is not available, but they are a lower-fat protein food than bacon rashers.

* Grated cheese goes further, regard 3 tbsp as a portion.

* Nuts are a fantastic source of protein, vitamins and minerals. You can have them as your protein by, for example, sprinkling some pine nuts into pasta, walnuts into a salad, or cashew nuts into a stir-fried veg and rice dish. Note that they are high in fat (healthy fats), so too many will pile on the pounds. Keep to 25 g (1 oz) of nuts or 2 tsp peanut butter a day.

* Choose canned beans in water rather than in sugar or salt.

* All peas, beans and lentils are nutritionally special foods, because as well as being packed with protein, they are also high in carbohydrates and low GI. They are an excellent choice as either your protein or carb food on your plate. If you choose them for protein, then remember to choose a carb to go with them. Likewise if you choose them to be your carb, then add a protein food.

🐦 *Protein is filling, but too much can put a strain on your kidneys, fill a quarter of your plate only with a lower-fat protein food*

Beans and Lentils	What it weighs	What it looks like
Baked beans, canned in tomato sauce	200 g	1 small can or ½ large can
Black gram, urad gram, dried, cooked	120 g (4½ oz)	3 serving spoons
Blackeye beans, dried, cooked	120 g (4½ oz)	3 serving spoons
Butter beans, dried, cooked	120 g (4½ oz)	3 serving spoons
Chickpeas, canned	120 g	½ large can
Chickpeas, whole, dried, cooked	120 g (4½ oz)	3 serving spoons
Reduced-fat hummus	½ pot	2 tablespoons
Chilli beans, canned	210 g	½ large can
Haricot beans, dried, cooked	120 g (4½ oz)	3 serving spoons
Haricot beans, dried, steamed	120 g (4½ oz)	3 serving spoons
Lentils, red, split, dried, cooked	120 g (4½ oz)	3 serving spoons
Mung beans, whole, dried, cooked	120 g (4½ oz)	3 serving spoons
Peas, fresh, steamed	75 g (3 oz)	3 serving spoons
Peas, frozen, steamed	75 g (3 oz)	3 serving spoons
Pigeon peas, whole, dried, cooked	120 g (4½ oz)	3 serving spoons
Pinto beans, dried, cooked	120 g (4½ oz)	3 serving spoons
Red kidney beans, canned	120 g	½ large can
Red kidney beans, dried, cooked	120 g (4½ oz)	3 serving spoons
Soya beans, dried, cooked	120 g (4½ oz)	3 serving spoons
Sweetcorn, kernels, canned, drained	75 g (3 oz)	2 rounded serving spoons

Sweetcorn kernels, frozen, steamed	75 g (3 oz)	2 rounded serving spoons
Sweetcorn on-the-cob, grilled		1 whole cob
Tesco Green Lentils	130 g	½ large can
Tesco Healthy Living Baked Beans	220 g	1 small can
Tesco Mixed Beans Italienne	150 g	1 small can

Eggs	What it looks like
Eggs, boiled	2 eggs
Eggs, fried in 1 tsp oil	2 eggs
Eggs, poached	2 eggs
Eggs, scrambled, with milk and 1 tsp oil	2 eggs
Omelette, plain, made with 1 tsp oil	2 eggs

Fish	What it looks like
Anchovies, drained	6 anchovies
Cockles	6 cockles
Cod, baked (can be in breadcrumbs)	1 fillet
Cod, grilled	1 fillet
Crab meat	2 tablespoons
Fish fingers, cod, grilled	4 fingers
Haddock, smoked	1 fillet
Haddock, steamed or grilled (can be in breadcrumbs)	1 fillet
Halibut, steamed or grilled	1 steak
Herring, grilled	2 fillets
Lemon sole, steamed or grilled	1 fillet

Lobster	2 tablespoons
Mackerel	1 fillet
Mussels	6 mussels
Oysters	12 oysters
Pilchards	2 pilchards
Plaice, steamed or grilled	1 fillet
Prawns	3 serving spoons
Salmon, pink, canned in brine, drained	200 g can, drained weight 150 g
Salmon, smoked	3 slices
Salmon, steamed or grilled	1 steak/fillet piece
Sardines, canned in brine, drained	4 sardines
Scallops, steamed	3 tablespoons
Shrimps	1 teacupful
Shrimps, canned in brine, drained	3 serving spoons
Trout, steamed or grilled	1 fillet
Tuna, canned in brine or water, drained	200 g can, drained weight 150 g

Meats	**What it looks like**
Bacon, gammon joint, lean only, cooked	150 g (5 oz) steak
Bacon rashers, lean, grilled	2 rashers
Beef, mince, cooked, lean, less than 10% fat	2 serving spoons
Beef, rump steak, lean, grilled	150 g (5 oz) steak
Beef sirloin joint, roasted, lean	3 slices
Beef stew, made with lean beef	2 serving spoons
Beefburgers, grilled	one 100 g (4 oz) beefburger

Chicken, breast chunks or strips	2 serving spoons
Chicken, breast, skinless, roasted	1 medium
Chicken, drumstick, skinless, dry-roasted	2 drumsticks
Chicken, leg, skinless, dry-roasted	1 medium
Chicken, roasted	3 slices
Chicken, thigh, skinless, dry-roasted	1 medium
Chicken, wing, skinless, roasted	4 wings
Duck, dry-roasted	3 slices
Ham	2 slices
Ham, wafer thin	6 slices
Kidney, lamb, sautéed	2 kidneys
Kidney, ox, stewed	3 tablespoons
Lamb, breast, roasted, lean	2 slices
Lamb, leg steaks, lean, grilled	150 g (5 oz) steak
Lamb, loin chops, grilled, lean	2 chops
Lamb, scrag and neck, lean only, stewed	2 serving spoons
Lamb, shanks	1 small shank
Liver, ox, stewed	3 tablespoons
Pork leg joint, dry-roasted	3 slices
Pork, loin chops, grilled, lean	1 chop
Rabbit, stewed	2 serving spoons
Turkey, cooked	2 slices
Turkey, cooked, wafer thin	6 slices
Turkey mince	2 serving spoons
Turkey, roasted	2 slices

Milk and Dairy	What it weighs	What it looks like
Cheese, Camembert	40 g (1½ oz)	
Cheese, Cheddar	25 g (1 oz)	2.5-cm (1-in) cube or equivalent to 2 jelly cubes
Cheese, Cheddar, half-fat	40 g (1½ oz)	
Cheese, Cheddar, strong, grated	25 g (1 oz)	3 level tablespoons
Cheese, Edam	40 g (1½ oz)	piece the size of 6 jelly cubes (half a block of raw jelly)
Cheese, feta	40 g (1½ oz)	
Cheese, Jarlsberg	40 g (1½ oz)	
Cheese, low-fat, soft (e.g. extra-light version of cream cheese)	50 g	¼ of tub
Cheese, medium-fat, soft (e.g. light version of cream cheese)	40 g (1½ oz)	1 mini tub (35 g) or ⅕ of 200 g tub
Cheese, Mini Babybel Light	40 g (1½ oz)	2 individual portions
Cheese, mozzarella	40 g (1½ oz)	⅓ of a ball
Cheese, ricotta	150 g	1 small tub
Cottage cheese, reduced-fat	200 g	1 large tub
Milk, semi- or skimmed	200 ml (7 fl oz)	full glass
Soya alternative to yoghurt	120 g	1 small pot
Yoghurt, diet	120 g	1 small pot
Yoghurt, Greek, sheep's	150 ml	1 small pot

Yoghurt, low-fat Greek style, natural	150 ml	1 small pot

Nuts	**What it weighs**	**What it looks like**
Almonds	15 g (½ oz)	10–12 almonds
Cashew nuts	15 g (½ oz)	10–12 cashews
Peanuts, dry roasted	25 g (1 oz)	1 pub pack or half 50 g pack
Peanuts, in shells	25 g (1 oz)	15 shells
Peanuts, roasted and salted	25 g (1 oz)	1 pub pack or half 50 g pack
Pecans	15 g (½ oz)	10 halves
Pine nuts	15 g (½ oz)	1 tablespoon
Walnuts	15 g (½ oz)	8 halves

Other Protein Foods	**What it weighs**	**What it looks like**
Tofu, cooked	150 g (5 oz)	10-cm (4-in) square piece
Quorn burgers, grilled		2 burgers
Quorn, pieces, as purchased		12 pieces

Protein recipes

Chunky Hummus – see page 145
Minted Peas – see page 153
Teriyaki Chicken Strippers – see page 157
Saucy Chops – see page 158
Pork Steaks with Creamy Mustard Sauce – see page 159
Scotch Eggs – see page 160
Lamb Cutlets with Tomato and Mint Sauce – see page 161

> ❧ *What you eat today will show tomorrow – choose wisely*

10 things to do with poultry

* Make your own chicken burgers by mixing minced chicken with a beaten egg, a handful of breadcrumbs, some grated onion, herbs and seasoning. Form into burger shapes and grill or bake.

* Pan-fry turkey escalopes in 1 tsp olive oil and garlic. Cook on both sides till brown.

* Marinade chicken wings in a mixture of 1–2 tsp olive oil, 2 tsp honey, 2 tsp coarse grain mustard, 1–2 tbsp soy sauce and barbecue sauce if desired. Bake in the oven until the juices run clear.

* Use up leftover chicken by mixing shredded cooked chicken with cooked rice and vegetables.

* Cook a skinless chicken breast under the grill. Thicken some cream of chicken soup with a little cornflour paste and serve this speedy sauce over the chicken.

* Cook diced chicken in our *Really Useful Curry Base* recipe (see page 172) and serve an Indian take-away at home.

* Stir-fry strips of chicken or turkey breast and add this to cooked pasta with a low-fat tomato-based pasta sauce.

* Bake chicken pieces on the bone, wrapped in foil, flavoured in a drizzle of olive oil, garlic, mixed dried herbs and lemon or orange juice.

✳ Fill half a pitta bread with leftover chicken and salad.

✳ Flavour chicken drumsticks with paprika powder, chilli sauce and honey and roast in the oven.

10 things to do with fish

✳ Coat a salmon fillet with a mixture of lemon juice, chopped coriander leaves, crushed ginger and seasoning. Cook in the oven or under the grill for 10 minutes.

✳ Pan-fry your favourite fish in 1 tsp olive oil and crushed garlic. Drizzle with 1 tbsp lemon juice and serve sizzling from the pan.

✳ Coat white fish in beaten egg and then in orange bread-crumbs. Place on a lightly greased baking tray. Spray with a few sprays of one-calorie spray oil and grill or bake.

✳ Make Mediterranean fish parcels with haddock, diced peppers, sliced tomatoes, a few olives and some fresh or dried oregano wrapped in foil pockets and baked.

✳ Mix some cooked mackerel with ricotta cheese, dried herbs and black pepper to make an instant mackerel pâté.

✳ Throw a handful of cooked prawns into your favourite pasta or rice dish. All you need is two veggies or salad to make up your V V P C.

✳ Mix canned tuna with diced peppers, red onion and sweet-corn dressed in low-fat yoghurt. An excellent wrap, pitta, baked potato or sandwich filling.

✳ Conjure up a speedy prawn cocktail: mix together low-fat Greek yoghurt with 1 tsp tomato purée and ground white pepper. Smother this over cooked prawns, on a bed of shredded lettuce and serve with lemon wedges and crunchy granary toast. This gives you one Protein, one Veggie and one Carb, so all you need to do is enjoy a fruity accompaniment to make up the V V P C.

✳ Go Chinese style by making a dressing of soy sauce, a few drops of sesame oil, crushed ginger and a little honey. Brush this over your favourite fish and bake or grill.

✳ Mix canned tuna with cooked pasta and some canned beans dressed in fat-free dressing for a speedy tuna and bean salad.

   🐌 *Fry less, grill more*

THE CARB PART

This is an extensive list of low-GI carbs, but if something you like isn't here, it's possible the GI is too high for this Plan or GI-testing hasn't been done on it yet, so we just don't know the GI value. If you do want a more extensive list, check out *The 10-Day Gi Diet* (see page 235).

✳ All beans and lentils count once a day as one of your five fruit and veg. These are rich in both carbs and protein and if you choose them as your protein, then choose another carb from the carb boxes.

✳ The amount you eat is important – it's not just about GI. The GiP system also looks at amounts, a bit like putting GI and good health all into one package. So look carefully at the portion sizes and keep to them to ensure you get results.

✳ The boxes may not include all the things you will eat – like the sauce on the pasta or a dressing on a salad. Check out the lower-fat trimmings section on page 92.

✳ You'll see some veggies in the carb section as they are high in starch. Other vegetables are not – you can find these on pages 65–6.

✳ Use your common sense. If you don't find what you're

looking for, say frozen soya beans, then think: it's a good food, rich in protein and carbs like other beans, I'll use it as either a carb or protein and keep to the portions as for other beans. If you don't find the bread you like, think: if it has seeds, weighs around the same as other breads, then count it as a carb like the other breads.

✳ To flavour bread, try yeast extract (e.g. Marmite), light soft cheese, mustard, a scraping of butter or a little low-fat spread.

🫘 *Carbs are good – go for slow carbs like the ones listed here*

Beans and Lentils	What it weighs	What it looks like
Adzuki beans, cooked	120 g (4½ oz)	3 serving spoons
Baked beans, canned in tomato sauce	200 g	1 small can or ½ large can
Black gram, urad gram, dried, cooked	120 g (4½ oz)	3 serving spoons
Blackeye beans, cooked	120 g (4½ oz)	3 serving spoons
Broad beans, canned or steamed	2 tbsp	½ large can
Butter beans, dried, cooked	120 g (4½ oz)	3 serving spoons
Chickpeas, canned	120 g	½ large can
Chickpeas, whole, dried, cooked	120 g (4½ oz)	3 serving spoons
Chilli beans, canned	210 g	½ large can
Haricot beans, dried, cooked	120 g (4½ oz)	3 serving spoons
Lentils, red, split, dried, cooked	120 g (4½ oz)	3 serving spoons

Mung beans, whole, dried, cooked	120 g (4½ oz)	3 serving spoons
Pigeon peas, whole, dried, cooked	120 g (4½ oz)	3 serving spoons
Pinto beans, dried, cooked	120 g (4½ oz)	3 serving spoons
Red kidney beans, canned	120 g	½ large can
Red kidney beans, dried, cooked	120 g (4½ oz)	3 serving spoons
Soya beans, cooked	120 g	3 serving spoons
Tesco Cannellini Beans	150 g	½ can
Tesco Flageolet Beans	150 g	½ can
Tesco Green Lentils	130 g	½ large can
Tesco Healthy Living Baked Beans	220 g	1 small can or ½ large can
Tesco Mixed Beans Italienne	150 g	½ large can

Remember if you choose beans or lentils as your carb, you will need to choose a non-beanie food as your protein.

Starchy Vegetables	What it weighs	What it looks like
5%-fat oven chips	150 g (5 oz)	2 heaped serving spoons
Jacket potato, no added fat	120 g (4½ oz)	a tennis ball – eat with low-GI veggies
New potatoes, boiled	150 g (5 oz)	4 new potatoes
New potatoes, canned, drained	150 g (5 oz)	4 new potatoes
Old potatoes, boiled	150 g (5 oz)	3 egg-size potatoes
Sweet potato, baked	150 g (5 oz)	1 small potato

	What it weighs	What it looks like
Sweet potato, boiled	150 g (5 oz)	mobile phone, 12.5 cm (5–6 in) long
Sweet potato, steamed or microwaved	150 g (5 oz)	1 small potato

Breads	What it weighs	What it looks like
Barley bread	80 g	2 slices
Burgen Oat Bran, Barley and Honey Bread	80 g	2 slices
Burgen Soya and Linseed Bread	80 g	2 slices
Chapatis, no fat on top	50 g	1 chapati
Granary bread	80 g	2 slices
M & S Count On Us Country Grain	50 g	2 slices
M & S Golden Wholemeal Soft	80 g	2 slices
M & S Oatmeal Soft Farmhouse	80 g	2 slices
M & S Seeded Soft Batch	80 g	2 slices
M & S Two in One Roll	60 g	1 roll
Mixed grain bread	80 g	2 slices
Pumpernickel bread	80 g	2 small slices
Sainsbury's pittas	30 g	1 mini pitta or ½ a large pitta
Warburtons All In One Bread	80 g	2 slices
Warburtons All In One White Sandwich Rolls	80 g	1 roll
Wheat tortillas	50 g	1 wrap

Pasta	What it weighs	What it looks like
Egg tagliatelle, cooked	100 g (4 oz)	5 tablespoons
Egg tagliatelle, dried	50 g (2 oz)	2 nests
Fettucini, egg, cooked	120 g (4½ oz)	5 tablespoons
Fettucini, egg, raw	50 g (2 oz)	handful of short fettucini about the thickness of a forefinger
Linguini, thick or thin, cooked	120 g (4½ oz)	5 tablespoons
Linguini, thick or thin, dried	50 g (2 oz)	handful of short linguini about the thickness of a forefinger
Macaroni, cooked	120 g (4½ oz)	5 tablespoons
Macaroni, dried	50 g (2 oz)	⅓ cupful
Noodles, instant, cooked	100 g (4 oz)	5 tablespoons
Noodles, instant, dried	60 g (2½ oz)	½ sheet of medium noodles
Noodles, rice, cooked	150 g (5 oz)	5 tablespoons
Noodles, rice, dried	50 g (2 oz)	handful of short noodles about the thickness of a forefinger
Pasta, plain, cooked	100 g (4 oz)	5 tablespoons
Pasta, plain, dried	50 g (2 oz)	⅓ cupful
Spaghetti, white or brown, cooked	120 g (4½ oz)	5 tablespoons
Spaghetti, white or brown, dried	50 g (2 oz)	handful of short spaghetti about the thickness of a forefinger

Tesco Fusilli Pasta Twists, cooked	150 g (5 oz)	5 tablespoons
Tesco Fusilli Pasta Twists, dried	50 g (2 oz)	1 cupful

Rice and Grains	What it weighs	What it looks like
Bulgur wheat, cooked	120 g (4½ oz)	6 heaped tablespoons
Bulgur wheat, raw	50 g (2 oz)	3 tablespoons
Couscous, cooked	100 g (4 oz)	1 cupful
Couscous, raw	40 g (1½ oz)	2 tablespoons
Rice, brown, boiled	150 g (5 oz)	2 serving spoons
Rice, white, basmati, boiled	150 g (5 oz)	2 serving spoons
Rice, white easy cook raw	50 g (2 oz)	½ cupful
Rice, white, easy cook, boiled	150 g (5 oz)	2 serving spoons
Rice, white, instant, boiled	150 g (5 oz)	2 serving spoons
Rice, white, polished, boiled	150 g (5 oz)	2 serving spoons
Rice, white, precooked, microwaved	150 g (5 oz)	2 serving spoons or ½ sachet

Soups* eaten with a slice of bread	What it weighs	What it looks like
Instant noodle soup	400 g (14 oz)	1 soup bowl (half a packet)
Lentil soup	400 g (14 oz)	1 soup bowl
Tomato soup, cream of, canned	400 g (14 oz)	1 soup bowl

* Note that any lower-fat soups are fine; they may not be listed here as they have not been tested for GI.

Some golden soup rules:

✳ If your soup is based mainly on a starchy carb like potato or parsnip, then you already have enough carb to meet the 'C' portion of your plate and you won't need the slice of bread.

✳ Chuck in your favourite veggies, fresh or frozen (keep them whole if you can) and add your protein (you could throw in some kidney beans or top with grated Cheddar).

✳ Generally, go for chunky soups rather than puréed ones as the mashing up disrupts the fibre and can raise the GI rating.

Sandwich lunch today?

It's not always possible or practical to have a plated meal – sometimes you just want to buy a sandwich and go. Keep to our basic rules of food choice, like going for seeded or grainy breads, lower-fat fillings such as tuna, chicken (in yoghurt or low fat dressing), hummus, lots of salad veg and no butter. Many sandwich bars are willing to customise choices – if you don't ask, you don't get! And, just to make life easier for healthy Hot Body seekers, many stores have now analysed the GI ratings of their popular sandwiches, so you can just buy, go and enjoy – with the knowledge that it's helping you keep to your Plan. Here are a few:

M & S Count on Us Chicken and Bacon Sandwich

M & S Count on Us Chicken and Balsamic Tomato Sandwich

M & S Count on Us Chicken No Mayo Sandwich

M & S Count on Us Ham Salad Sandwich

M & S Count on Us Hoisin Duck Wrap

M & S Count on Us Nacho Chicken Wrap

M & S Eat Well Chicken and Sweetcorn Sandwich

M & S Eat Well Chicken Salad Sandwich

M & S Eat Well Coronation Chicken Sandwich

M & S Eat Well Free Range Egg and Ham Sandwich

M & S Eat Well Free Range Egg and Prawn Sandwich

M & S Eat Well Free Range Egg and Watercress

M & S Eat Well Omega-3 Egg Sandwich

M & S Eat Well Poached Salmon and Watercress Sandwich

M & S Eat Well Prawn Mayonnaise Sandwich

M & S Eat Well Rare Roast Beef and Horseradish Sandwich

M & S Eat Well Salmon and Cucumber Sandwich

M & S Eat Well Southern Fried Chicken Wrap

M & S Eat Well Tuna and Cucumber Sandwich

M & S Eat Well Tuna and Sweetcorn Sandwich

Sainsbury's Be Good to Yourself Egg and Cress Sandwich

Sainsbury's Be Good To Yourself Tuna and Cucumber Sandwich

And if it's not a sandwich….

M & S Count on Us Mini Tuna Layer – add one wholemeal mini pitta

M & S Count on Us Tuna Salad – add your carb, e.g. Two in One Roll

M & S Eat Well Spiced Chicken with Eat Well Pomegranate Rice

2 packets M & S Eat Well Sushi to Snack

M & S Eat Well Tuna with Oriental Edamame Bean Salad

Remember to add:

✳ Your extra veg portion (e.g. a salad dressed in fat-free dressing), and

✳ 1 piece of fruit or 1 glass of unsweetened fruit juice

Ready Meals

With the best will in the world, sometimes you just can't be bothered with cooking, and a ready meal on occasions is fine. It all depends on what you're choosing and what you team it up with. Aim to get to the V V P C plate by adding lots of steamed veg or salads and remember to end your meal with a piece of fruit. Here are some GiP-counted ready meal ideas:

M & S Count On Us Chilli Tomato Chicken and Rice

M & S Count On Us King Prawn Pappardelle

M & S Count On Us King Prawn Pasta

M & S Count On Us Paella

M & S Count On Us Sweet Paprika Chicken with Patatas Bravas

M & S Count On Us Tomato and Basil Pasta

M & S Eat Well Butternut Squash Risotto (risotto rice is generally high GI, but these dishes are low GI because of other added ingredients)

M & S Eat Well Chicken and Asparagus Risotto

M & S Eat Well Harrissa Chicken with Couscous

M & S Eat Well Jambalaya

M & S Eat Well King Prawn with Coriander Couscous

M & S Eat Well Pasta with Cherry Tomatoes, Spinach and Pine Nuts

M & S Eat Well Pasta with Feta Cheese and Slow Roasted Tomatoes

M & S Eat Well Pasta with Poached Scottish Salmon

M & S Eat Well Roasted Red Onion and Goats' Cheese Pappardelle

2 Tesco Chicken Fajitas (½ pack of 4)

Tesco Chicken Szechuan

Tesco Cumberland Fish Bake (¼ pack)

Tesco Healthy Living Chicken Chow Mein

Tesco Healthy Living Lasagne

Tesco Finest Lasagne (½ pack)

Tesco Mushroom burger – add a seeded bap and salad

Tesco Penne Mozzarella Bake

And when you fancy a curry, remember to team this up with steamed basmati rice (50 g/2 oz dried weight or 2 serving spoons, 150 g/5 oz cooked) and a side salad:

M & S Eat Well Andhra Lamb Curry

M & S Eat Well Keralan Beef

M & S Eat Well Keralan King Prawn Curry (serves 2)

M & S Eat Well Malabar Fish Curry

NOTE: We have only included ready meals from these supermarkets because we have the GI and calorie data for these foods. This doesn't mean that you can't choose a ready meal from another store. Simply choose the supermarket's healthier versions, get a sense for lower-GI ingredients (like pasta, beans, lentils and couscous) and compare labels for fat and calories.

Carb Recipes

Fasta Pasta – see page 147

Veggie Bulgur Wheat – see page 150

Chinese Noodle and Baby Corn Soup – see page 155

Fruity Bulgur with Cashew Nuts – see page 156

    🍂 *Avoid TV dinners and snacks*

What's not here and why...

Okay, so you love parsnips and butternut squash and are still hunting for them on this list. Well, they are great foods: filling and fibrous. The reason why they are not listed is because they make your blood sugar go up quickly. GI research is based on single foods and when you eat parsnips or indeed a jacket potato on its own, it is quickly digested releasing its sugar into your blood stream very quickly (similar to white bread). In the real world we eat them with stuff (vegetables, cheese and so on) – and this affects the GI. But there is no data on jacket potatoes with fillings (or parsnips with other veggies). However, we appreciate that a baked potato is a classic warming food for people watching their waistline, so we have included it in the above list, but note that it needs to be eaten with low-GI accompaniments like sweetcorn or baked beans to get your blood sugar working for you.

Similarly, snack foods such as rice cakes and popcorn can make your blood sugar rise very quickly. The difference here is that these foods are more likely to be eaten on their own rather than as part of a meal, so other parts of the meal won't be able to slow down your blood sugar rise. In terms of GI, we don't recommend them, unless of course you're having them with low-GI accompaniments (such as reduced-fat hummus or peanut butter on the rice cakes). However, in terms of calories, they are perfectly acceptable as part of a weight-watching lifestyle.

The Hot Body Plan, remember, is about common sense. If you fancy a food that you know is healthy yet it's not listed here, and you're going to have it with a low-fat, low-GI accompaniment or filling, then go for it! Try to keep to the lists most of the time but you will at times have to make choices using your own initiative – and all this helps you to learn new tricks.

LOWER-FAT TRIMMINGS
* Salads – choose low-fat (3–5 per cent fat) or fat-free dressing, either bought, made up (lemon juice and black pepper is simple yet tasty) or try out one of our GiP-free dressing recipes (page 167).

✻ Pasta – choose a tomato-based sauce as it's lower in fat than creamy or cheesy ones. Or try out our pasta sauce recipe (see page 173) to jazz up any type of pasta.

✻ Clear soups belong in the veggie section and so are free. Ready to eat or homemade, they can be a welcome change from veggie crudités, especially in cold weather. Others, like lentil or pea soup, offer protein, so team them up with a carb such as some granary bread for a main meal. Soups store well in the fridge or freezer, so cook up a large saucepan full to keep you going for a while!

FREE FOODS

Artificial sweeteners

Chilli sauce

Fat-free horseradish sauce

Herbs, fresh or dried

Jelly

Mustard

Oil, spray oil

Pepper

Salad dressing

Salt (don't overdo it for health reasons!)

Salt substitutes

Soy sauce (try reduced-salt types)

Spices, fresh (e.g. garlic, ginger, chilli)

Spices, ground (e.g. paprika, chilli powder, curry powder)

Spices, whole (e.g. cumin seeds, coriander seeds, caraway seeds)

Stock cube

Sugar-free drinks

Sugar-free mint sauce

Tomato purée

Vinegar (rice, balsamic, malt, wine)

Worcestershire sauce

Yeast extracts and Bovril (no need to add salt if used in cooking, as
they're quite salty)

Free Dressings and Sauce Recipes

Coriander and Mint Chutney – see page 167
Balsamic and Honey Dressing – see page 168
Minty Moments – see page 168
Shai's Salsa – see page 169
Really Useful Curry Base – see page 172

MIXED DISHES AND THE HOT BODY PLAN

What about foods that are a mixture of proteins and carbs –
such as pizza or lasagne? Well, this Plan is about using your
common sense. If you fancy pizza, make sure you go for a thin-
based one with less cheese and more veggies – and of course
add heaps of salad on the side. You won't need the garlic bread
or you'll be adding too many carbs (remember V V P C).

Similarly, if you choose lasagne, imagine splitting the pasta
layers from the meat and cheese – does your portion size look
roughly like it would fit into the V V P C plate quarters? If not,
have less of the lasagne and more of the veggies and salads.

Ready meals and convenience foods aren't out of bounds,
you know. The foods and meals in this chapter have been tested
for their GI value, so you can choose these on occasions. Others

will be appropriate but because they haven't been tested for GI, we don't know what their value would be in the GiP System. Remember that ready meals and takeaways are unlikely to provide you with the balanced range of nutrients you can achieve in home-made meals, but there are times when you need to opt for convenience. Simply choose the foods from this chapter and add lots of veggies and salad to keep to the V V P C rule.

SNACK TIME?

In between meals, healthy snacks help to keep your hunger at bay and also steady your blood-sugar levels. Choose a piece of fruit, diet yoghurt, fruit mini-drink (such as a Knorr Vie Shot or M & S Eat Well Fresh Fruit in a Bottle – Apple and Kiwi, or Tesco Probiotic Cranberry or Orange Drink), or a handful of dried fruit.

If you're feeling really hungry and haven't had any nuts that day, then munch on 25 g (I oz) – a small handful – of your favourite nuts, ideally unsalted, or go for 10 shells of peanuts. Opening the shells means they take longer to eat!

And if you just fancy a hot cuppa and a biscuit, then opt for one or two semi-sweet biscuits like Rich Tea or Marie, or a couple of oat cakes.

WHAT TO ADD TO MAKE UP YOUR V V P C

Bacon rashers, back, grilled	3 rashers	V V C
Bacon rashers, middle, grilled	3 rashers	V V C
Beans, mung, green, gram, cooked dahl	I teacupful	V V C

Beefburgers, chilled/frozen, grilled	1 beefburger	V V C
Chicken nuggets, takeaway	6 nuggets	V V C
Chicken, stir-fried with steamed rice and vegetables, frozen	ready meal portion	V
Indian Dhokra	4 small pieces	V V P
Lamb/beef hot pot with potatoes, chilled/frozen	ready meal portion	V V
Macaroni cheese, lower-fat	2 serving spoons	V V
Ravioli, meat	12 ravioli	V V
Sainsbury's Be Good To Yourself Chicken Tikka Masala and Rice	per pack	V V
Sainsbury's Be Good To Yourself Egg and Cress Sandwich	whole pack	V V
Sainsbury's Be Good To Yourself Tuna and Cucumber Sandwich	whole pack	V V
Sushi (fish)	6 mini	V V
Takeaway pizza, cheese and tomato, deep pan	⅓ of a medium (23-cm/9-in diameter) or ⅛ of a large (30-cm/ 12-in diameter)	V V
Takeaway pizza, cheese and tomato, thin base	⅓ of a medium (23-cm/9-in diameter) or ⅛ of a large (30-cm/ 12-in diameter)	V V
Takeaway pizza, vegetarian	⅓ of a medium (23-cm/9-in diameter) or ⅛ of a large (30-cm/ 12-in diameter)	V V
Tesco Chicken Szechuan	350 g	V V C

Tesco Cumberland Fish Bake	237.5 g (¼ pack)	V V
Tesco Healthy Living Chicken Chow Mein	450 g	V V
Tesco Healthy Living Lasagne	340 g	V V
Tesco Mushroom Burger	87.5 g (½ pack)	V P C
Tesco Penne Mozzarella Bake	340 g	V V
Tesco Roasted Winter Vegetables	200 g (½ pack)	P C
Tortellini, cheese	12 tortellini	V V
Vine leaves, stuffed with rice	8 medium vine leaves	V P

And as for recipes, there is a host of tasty delights in our recipe chapter. Here are some of the choices you can have that offer you the perfect V V P C combinations:

Recipes	What to add to make VVPC	Serving suggestion
10-minute Trout with Exotic Seeds	V V C	serving of Veggie Bulgur Wheat (see page 150), mixed leaf salad
Asparagus Anticipation	V P C	roasted chicken breast, 2 serving spoons basmati rice, grilled aubergines
Cabbage with Fennel Seeds	P C	2 serving spoons beef stew, made with lean beef, 4 new potatoes
Chunky Hummus	V V C	pitta strips (half a pitta), carrot sticks, green salad

Fasta Pasta	negligible	side salad
Guacamole with Bite	V P C	crisp salad, 40 g (1½ oz) feta cheese, 1 wheat tortilla
Honeyed Mange Tout	V P C	1 small lamb shank, small baked sweet potato, cauliflower
Lamb Cutlets with Tomato and Mint Sauce	V C	courgettes, cupful of couscous cooked in lamb stock
Minted Peas	V P C	fillet of cod baked in breadcrumbs, grilled tomatoes, crusty granary bread
Pork Steaks with Creamy Mustard Sauce	V V C	4 new potatoes, grilled mushrooms followed by a tangy apple
Posh Fish Fingers with Tartare Sauce	V V C	heaped serving spoon 5%-fat oven chips, 2–3 tbsp peas, 2 grilled tomatoes
Saucy Chops	V V C	4 new potatoes in their skins, mange tout, baby sweetcorn
Thai Baby Corn and Mange Tout with Crushed Peanuts	C	½ sheet dried noodles, boiled
Tiger Prawns with Creamy Dipping Sauce	V V C	2 slices soya and linseed toast topped with grilled mushrooms, watercress salad

| Veggie Bulgur Wheat | P | 8 walnut halves, chopped and scattered on top |
| Teriyaki Chicken Strippers | V V C | tortilla wrap with crunchy fresh salad vegetables |

HOW DOES THIS MAKE V V P C?

Saucy Chops

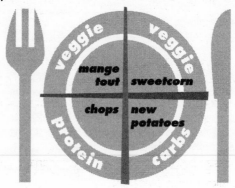

Minted Peas

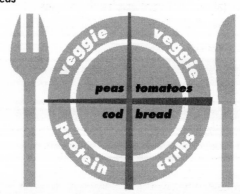

3. NOW CHOOSE YOUR FRUIT

Get into the habit of completing your meal with a piece of fruit, especially if you feel you have not quite managed your full veggie portions. Most fruit are generally low in GI and packed with antioxidants and fibre, just like most veg. We know, you've heard it before − eat five a day. Despite the fact that the Food Standards Agency and British Dietetic Association have run campaigns on promoting five fruit and vegetables a day, current intakes in the UK are still averaging around two portions. Many people are confused by exactly what a portion of fruit is. Here are some examples:

One portion of any fruit or vegetable weighs 80 g (3 oz) − that is the weight of the edible bit, so a whole apple may weigh around 100 g (4 oz). A 75 g (3 oz) portion of lettuce is roughly equivalent to a cereal bowlful and 75 g (3 oz) of cooked vegetables is roughly 3 tablespoons.

✳ Medium-size piece of fruit, e.g. apple, banana, orange
✳ 1 large slice melon, pineapple
✳ 2 plums, apricots, satsumas, kiwi
✳ Handful (about a dozen) grapes or cherries
✳ 3 tbsp fresh fruit salad or canned fruit in natural juice
✳ Half a grapefruit
✳ Half an avocado
✳ 1 tbsp dried fruit e.g. raisins, apricots
✳ 1 glass (150 ml/5 fl oz) unsweetened fresh fruit juice (counts only once as one of your five a day; have fruit juice as part of a meal rather than in between meals)

… And on days when you just don't feel like fruit − go for a scoop of lower-fat ice cream, or a diet yoghurt or check out our recipes on pages 174–7.

You can choose to have a piece of fruit after your V V P C meal or, if you prefer, have a piece of fruit instead of one of your portions of vegetables or salad.

> ঽ➤ *A piece of fruit can count as one of your veggie quarters*

FRUITY RECIPES
Red Fruit Compote – see page 174
Melon and Raspberry with Mint – see page 175
Warm Bananas with Orange – see page 176
Lychees with Pistachio – see page 177
Grilled Oranges – see page 177

HAVING A SNACK ATTACK?

This plan is based on eating little and often, not going hungry, and allowing yourself treats too. Healthy snacks can be good for your mental performance; they're helpful in keeping you alert throughout the day. With GI eating, they can be your best friends as they help you to keep your blood sugar steady. What's more, they can positively help you watch that waistline since a feeling of fullness means you're less likely to raid the fridge as soon as you get home.

Be it mid-morning, mid-afternoon or even – occasionally – late evening, enjoy one of our snacks. The Hot Body Plan recommends two light snacks per day, so choose away.

WARM 'N' CUDDLY

Bowl of canned cream of tomato soup
Bowl of instant noodle soup (use ½ packet)
Bowl of lentil soup (less mushy means lower GI)
Mug of reduced-fat hot chocolate
Mug of latte made with skimmed milk, no sugar (use a sweet-
ener if you like)

SWEET STUFF

Low-fat diet yoghurt
150 ml (5 fl oz) low-fat Greek style, natural yoghurt
Small pot of reduced-fat mousse (100 calories or less)
Small pot of soya alternative to yoghurt

DRINKS

Glass of drinking yoghurt (choose reduced-fat variety if possible)
Glass of flavoured milkshake, reduced-fat
Tesco Probiotic Orange or Cranberry Drink
Knorr Vie Shot Orange, Banana or Carrot
200 ml (7 fl oz) Chocolate Nesquik made with skimmed or
semi-skimmed milk
innocent Kids Oranges, Mangoes and Pineapples, 180 ml carton
innocent Strawberries and Bananas, 150 ml (5 fl oz) glass
innocent Mangoes and Passionfruit, 150 ml (5 fl oz) glass

MUNCHY SNACKS (CHOOSE NUTS ONLY
ONCE A DAY)

Half a large can of fruit, canned in juice or water
1 piece of fruit
1 handful (about a dozen) grapes
4 dried dates or apricots

1 handful (1 tbsp) sultanas

Half an avocado with lemon and black pepper

Around 20 olives, drained (you could add a few pickled onions or gherkins)

1 handful (25 g/1 oz) roasted soya nuts

10 almonds

10 peanuts in shells (they take longer to eat!)

8–10 cashews

6 pecan halves

5 walnut halves

Carrot sticks with low-fat natural yoghurt (try our *Cucumber Raita Dip*, page 171)

Cucumber with 2 tbsp guacamole (try the *Guacamole with Bite*, page 146)

TEATIME SNACKS

1 oatcake

1 Jacob's Essentials – wholewheat crackers with sesame seeds and rosemary

1 Rich Tea biscuit

1 cream cracker with ricotta cheese and cracked black pepper

1 rye crispbread, topped with cottage cheese or very low-fat soft cheese

2 wholemeal crackers

1 cracker with 1 tsp Nutella hazelnut spread

COLD YET FILLING

Warburtons All In One White Sandwich Roll with a little ricotta cheese

Small can baked beans, in tomato sauce

Half a can of chick peas, flavoured with Tabasco and lemon juice

Half a can of Tesco Mixed Beans Italienne

Small tub of cottage cheese (any flavour, throw in some diced
    cucumber if you like)
1 Mini Babybel Light
Small can drained tuna mixed with 1 tbsp canned sweetcorn
Light salad dressed in fat-free dressing

FREE SNACK ATTACK BOX – HAVE AS OFTEN AS YOU LIKE

Simply throw together any combination of the following: courgette sticks, cucumber sticks, baby gherkins, radishes, cherry
tomatoes, celery, baby sweetcorn, sugar snap peas, pickled
onions, peppers, water chestnuts.

TREAT TIME – HAVE NO MORE THAN FOUR A WEEK – WHEN ONLY A TREAT WILL DO!

This list contains items that have not been GI-tested so are not
strictly analysed within the GiP System. However, they contain
around 100 calories each and, after all, it's treat time! Have them
on four occasions, instead of one of your usual snacks.

Chocolate, milk	1 treat-size bar (15 g)
Chocolate, white	1 treat-size bar (13 g)
Snickers bar	1 fun-size bar (19 g)
Twix	1 mini Twix (21 g)
Go Lower bar	1 34 g bar
Mars bar	1 fun-size bar (19 g)
Small cereal bar, 100 calorie type	
Any 2 fresh fruits	
1 chocolate biscuit	
Mini chocolate Swiss roll	

Small bag Twiglets, Skips or Quavers

2 ginger nuts or jaffa cakes

Hot chocolate drink (sachet) made with skimmed milk

Thick slice of garlic bread

Slice of fruit loaf

200 g pot light fruit yoghurt (very low-fat and sugar free)

I medium slice of seeded bread with low-fat spread and Marmite

2-finger KitKat

I Scotch pancake

I heaped serving spoon (60 g/2½ oz) oven chips, approximately 5% fat

---

WHAT ABOUT OTHER SUPERMARKETS?

We are not recommending you shop in the listed supermarkets only or you only buy the featured brands. The reason for high-lighting these choices is that we have been able to get GI data directly from the retailers and manufacturers so we can incorporate them into our GiP System, doing all the calculations for you to use the foods as part of the V V P C strategy. If you find other brands of the same basic foods, give them a try. Although we can't be sure they will be low GI, you will find it useful to compare labels for fat, sugar and calories. That way you are better able to make an informed choice.

> 🐚 *Keeping to the V V P C will help you to reduce your calories and eat well, whichever brand you use*

FAMILY FOODS

Since this isn't a diet, the whole family can join in your healthy way of eating. The only thing that will need to change is the portion size for family members not watching their weight, and of course, you will need to make sure that growing kids get enough fat and protein to give them the calories they need for growth.

HERE ARE SOME TIPS:

✳ Everyone can benefit from eating the V V P C way. The variety of colours provides important nutrients.

✳ Kids will need bigger portions in terms of protein and carbs, and you might want to add a knob of butter or 1 tsp olive oil to their veg if they are not overweight, as this adds valuable calories for growth. A child's plate is best divided differently – more like ⅓ each for Veggies, Protein and Carbs (V P C). Snacks too are important for younger children to maintain energy levels and concentration. For this reason, some primary schools allow the children to bring in fruit for morning break. Teenagers can be encouraged into eating more fruit and veg by reminding them that these are good for healthy skin and hair, and so general good looks!

✳ Men can enjoy the GiP way of eating too – research shows that low-GI eating can help reduce the risk of heart disease. Get your man to slim and trim with you – he may need larger portion sizes, but the basic meals can be the same.

HOT BODY TRIALS

We've been very fortunate to have some volunteers try out the Hot Body Plan before you do, to provide us with valuable feedback. Here's a selection of some of their views:

'The only time I felt hungry on this Plan was when I missed a snack. I found it so easy to remember to fill half my plate with veg – no calorie counting like other diets I've been on. Though I didn't keep rigidly to the plan, I lost almost 1 kg (2 lb) by the end of the week. I prefer the slow, steady approach as I know it will help me keep it off.' Felicity

'Finally a "diet" that is for people like me – lazy, unimaginative in cooking, a real can't-cook-won't-cook person, not a lot of willpower or motivation. I feel that this "Hot Body Plan" is literally spoon-feeding me just the way I like. No counting, no weighing, no measuring – it's all done for me and all I have to do is decide which combination I want to go for – easy peasy! I feel that I can carry on with this long term. I lost ½ kg (1lb) in just over a week.' Nafisha

'Once I had made out a two-day meal planner I was away! I'm proud of myself for having followed the diet pretty much to the letter as I'm not usually that good. I do get hungry and am always ready for my next meal or snack – just shows you how we get used to eating so much! Lost 1 kg (2 lb) in a week, which I was supposed to. I now realise it's better to lose small and often, so if I lose the same next week, I'll be feeling smug.' Sue

And some quick tips…

'I brush my teeth after my evening meal and this leaves me with such a fresh feeling that I really don't need to corrupt my mouth with anything more. I'm also too lazy to brush my teeth again, so this stops me from nibbling.' Lorraine

'I love chocolate and there are times when I can't prevent myself from thinking about it. My friend bought me a chocolate-scented candle, and I light it whenever those chocolate messages enter my brain. Guess what? The beautiful aroma is enough to satisfy my craving!'

Marta

'When you have a craving, it really helps to drink some water and wait for about 20 minutes – just distract yourself. Often you'll find that the craving has gone and you'll feel really proud of yourself.'

Nigel

PUTTING IT ALL TOGETHER

Here is that handy checklist again to remind you of what you need to do every day.

Every day choose:	
Breakfast	1 from list
Free veggies	4 servings
Protein portions	2 servings
Carb portions	2 servings
Fruit	2 servings, 1 as part of each main meal
Snacks	2, at least 1 being fruit
Milk, semi- or skimmed	200 ml (7 fl oz) for beverages
Dairy foods	Make sure that as well as your milk above, you include two lower-fat dairy based foods from the protein portions, breakfasts or snacks

Water, tea, coffee, low-calorie squash, low-calorie flavoured waters	6–8 cups or glasses a day
And get physical!	Two 10-minute bursts of moderate intensity activity

At the end of this chapter, you will find a meal planner to help you decide how you are going to put together your first week's meals. Once you get used to it, this way of eating will become second nature.

So for each day, your goal is to choose one breakfast, two to three snacks and a veggie veggie protein carb and fruit choice for each main meal. In addition, here are some top tips to help you keep to the more nutritious choices.

✳ Make sure you have at least five portions of fruit and veggies each day. In fact, you'll probably find you're having more than this if you keep to the choices recommended.

✳ You need three average servings of calcium each day for healthy bones. So make sure you have your daily allowance of milk as well as two other servings of low-fat calcium foods. Examples of servings include a pot of yoghurt, 25 g (1 oz) of cheese, a glass of milk, or soya alternatives to these dairy products. If you do not take milk in your drinks then have an extra serving, such as low-fat soft cheese, to make three.

✳ Drink lots of water in between meals. Remember that tea, coffee, flavoured waters, unsweetened fruit juice and low-calorie squash all count towards your daily recommended fluid intake of 6–8 glasses a day. Note that 150 ml (5 fl oz) fruit juice only counts once a day towards your five a day fruit and vegetable recommendation. Try to have juice with meals rather than in between meals, as this can slow down the rise in blood sugar.

✳ The Plan is roughly equivalent to 1400–1500 calories per day. This may seem like a lot of calories compared to other diets you've been on, but there is evidence to suggest that people do better in the long term on slightly more calories. So enjoy with a clear conscience!

Remember to keep to the alcohol recommendations on page 115. Aim for no more than seven units of alcohol a week and it's best to have two or three drink-free days each week. But remember that alcohol lowers your blood-sugar levels and may leave you feeling hungry.

HOT TIPS FOR HEALTHY EATING HABITS

Eating consciously, and savouring each mouthful, go a long way towards healthy eating. Whatever your circumstances, whether you live on your own, or share your household, here are some suggestions to make one of life's pleasurable pastimes, even more enjoyable. You may wish to keep a food diary, too.

✳ Shop when you've eaten, so you'll ignore the temptation to buy all sorts of extras. Make a shopping list and stick to it.

✳ Watch out for ever-increasing portion sizes on ready meals and snacks such as sandwiches, crisps and chocolate bars. Just switching from a standard bag of crisps to a large bag would cause up to 6 kg (14 lb) weight gain over a year without you changing anything else!

✳ Canned foods such as fruit, vegetables, pulses and fish can be useful. Look for those labelled 'reduced salt' or 'no added salt'.

✳ Remember dried and frozen foods too – often just as nutritious and more convenient if you don't shop every day.

✳ Put distractions on hold when eating, this includes reading, watching TV or DVDs. Choose calming and enjoyable music instead.

✳ Spend time appreciating your food – the longer the better.

✳ Directly after your meal, give yourself a few moments before moving on to the next task on the 'to do' list.

✳ Size does count! Select your appropriate serving, not necessarily the whole dish or bowl.

✳ Even if you're eating alone, make it a special occasion and set the table invitingly for one – you are worth it!

✳ Food can be a seductive experience when each mouthful is appreciated, S-L-O-W-L-Y.

✳ Using your awareness after each bite will allow your body to regulate the hunger scale, consciously. Stop when your body registers it's full.

✳ Drink water with your meal – we often mistake thirst for hunger, so quenching your thirst could help you to recognise your hunger cues more effectively.

If you are a 'super person' – and eating is something that needs to be fitted in among the other 50 things in your diary for the day – try these:

✳ Share one meal a day with the rest of the family. Research suggests that children can benefit from this experience, both in terms of social interaction and prevention of bad eating habits.

✳ Use your creativity and play with variety while keeping the meal simple yet nutritious. Jazzing up a salad with a few toasted pine nuts or garnishing the fish with some char-grilled red peppers can give you a better taste sensation.

✳ Make it a family affair and share the chores of clearing or washing after allowing the food to settle.

✳ If the kids go to war over the greens, you might lose the will to live by the time the issue has been resolved! Meal times are to be enjoyed, so serve up some healthy, simple choices.

And, when dining out:

✳ Never arrive at the restaurant starving! Eat a light snack beforehand. Sounds mad but it will help you to avoid guzzling down the bread like a vacuum cleaner!

✳ Most pasta has a low GI, but it's the sauces served with it that can be laden with fat and calories. Order pasta with a fresh tomato sauce, which tends to be lower in fat than cream-based sauces, and say 'no' to the Parmesan cheese. Ask for your plate to be filled half with a crunchy selection of mixed salad leaves and half with the pasta of your choice (V V P C in action!).

✳ Deep-pan pizza bases are likely to have a higher GI and, because they have more carbs, the GiP value will be high too. So go for a thin-based pizza with masses of low-GI vegetable toppings. Steer clear of extra cheese and processed pepperoni.

✳ Ask for a GiP-free side salad with your meal. As for the dress-ing, balsamic vinegar or a squeeze of lemon juice and a sprin-kling of herbs can do the trick. Or ask for dressing on the side and neatly put it out of sight and temptation when it arrives.

✳ If you are having a grilled meat or chicken dish, ask for the sauce 'on the side' so you have control as to how much you eat, even better go without! Ask for unbuttered vegetables and boiled new potatoes in their skin.

✳ Ask for what you want – you're paying!

✳ Alcohol – flick to page 119 for our hot tips.

✳ Put your cutlery down between mouthfuls – chat more, drink more water, taste more.

✳ If you're tempted by the dessert menu, make a beeline for those with fruit and plain ice cream. Remember they may still be huge portions, so ask for two spoons and get up close and personal with your dinner date.

7-DAY MEAL PLANNER

Enlarge and photocopy the meal planner on page 114 or scan it into a computer and run off as many copies as you need. Then just jot down your planned food choices for the next week in the boxes as shown.

AND FINALLY...

✳ Carbs are not the enemy. Choosing low-GI carbs may actually help reduce the risk of diabetes and heart disease. Just keep to the advised portion sizes.

✳ Opt for fruit rather than fruit juice. You get more fibre and a lower-GI because your body has to work harder to break down the whole fruit.

✳ When choosing soup, go for those with whole beans and lentils. When choosing bread, go for bread with bits in it such as seeds and grains. When choosing vegetables, go for those that are whole rather than puréed.

✳ Wheat tortillas tend to have a lower GI then many breads. They make a great alternative to a lunchtime sandwich.

✳ Chew sugar-free gum when you feel peckish.

✳ Italians have found a way to make beans more digestible. It is said that they always cook beans with parsley to minimise any digestive discomfort.

* Hydrogenated or trans-fats are synthetically made and are thought to be more harmful than saturated fat. You find these in biscuits, cakes, pastries and many other processed foods.

* Watching your calories in small ways can make a big difference. The GiP System automatically helps you to do this. All you need to do is cut down by 500 calories a day and you will lose a pound of fat a week.

* Low energy levels? Choose a multigrain bread, apples, oranges, pears or a handful of dried apricots. The B vitamins and the low-GI effect will help to convert your blood sugar into slow steady energy for your body.

* You may think of beans as vegetables, but they are also packed with plant protein and carbs. They really belong to the starch or protein part of your V V P C plate. So, if you're having grilled fish fingers as your protein, you could have baked beans as your carb.

* Make your own fish fingers with some cod or salmon cut into finger-size portions. Dip into an egg white and then roll in a bowl of breadcrumbs. You could stick these in the freezer and simply bake in the oven when needed. They are lower in salt and far more nutritious than bought fish fingers.

* Lentils and bulgur wheat make a fantastic low-GI alternative to potatoes or rice.

* High in carbs, fibre, vitamins and minerals, wholegrain foods are associated with a reduced risk of coronary heart disease when eaten as part of a healthy balanced diet. Wholegrain foods can also help to reduce the risk of several types of chronic illness, such as stroke, certain types of cancer and type 2 diabetes.

	Day 1	Day 2	Day 3	Day 4	Day 5	Day 6	Day 7
Breakfast							
Mid-morning snack							
Lunch							
Veggie 1							
Veggie 2							
Carb							
Protein							
Fruit							
Mid-afternoon snack							
Evening meal							
Veggie 1							
Veggie 2							
Carb							
Protein							
Fruit							
Milk for drinks or high calcium alternative							
My 2 other calcium containing foods will be							
My 6–8 cups or glasses of fluid will be							

CHAPTER FIVE: FANCY A DRINK?

Having the occasional drink is fine, both in terms of your weight and your health, but when you drink above safe limits, that's when the calories go up and you are at greater risk of various health problems such as liver disease and cancer.

KNOW YOUR UNITS

The recommendations on safe alcohol intake are based upon how long it takes your body to metabolise alcohol. It is estimated that the average healthy adult body breaks down 10 ml (⅓ fl oz) of pure alcohol per hour. As a result, the UK 'unit' of alcohol has been set at around 10 ml (⅓ fl oz) of pure alcohol. The government advises that women drink less than two to three units per day and men drink a maximum of four units per day – it's better to drink less – with two to three alcohol-free days each week.

Alcohol by volume and serving sizes have gone up in recent years – and if you're friends with the barman, you may be getting more units per glass than you think! Overleaf is a summary of average units in common drinks.

Pint of ale/beer (4 per cent ABV)	just over 2 units
Pint of lager (5 per cent ABV)	nearly 3 units
440 ml can of lager (5 per cent ABV)	just over 2 units
Large 250 ml (8 fl oz) glass of wine (13 per cent ABV)	just over 3 units
Medium 175 ml (6 fl oz) glass of wine (13 per cent ABV)	just over 2 units
Small 125 ml (4 fl oz) glass of wine (9 per cent ABV)	just over 1 unit
Standard 175 ml (6 fl oz) glass of champagne (12 per cent ABV)	2 units
275 ml alcopop (5 per cent)	1½ units
Single measure of spirits (40 per cent ABV)	1 unit
(ABV – Alcohol by Volume)	

THE GREY AREAS

THE ALCOHOL CONTENT OF WINES

The alcohol content of wines has increased since the government set out its recommendations. One unit of alcohol used to be 125 ml (4 fl oz) of a wine that contained 8 per cent of alcohol by volume (ABV). Today a lot of wines sold may contain 13 per cent ABV and new world wines tend to have a higher alcohol content due to hotter climates. Alcohol content makes a big difference to the amount of units you may drink at any one time. For example, a standard glass of 13 per cent ABV wine contains 2.1 units compared to 1.6 units in a standard glass of 9 per cent ABV. To monitor how much you are drinking read the labels on your wine bottles to gauge the wine strength, or ask your bartender for the alcohol content of the wine. It may be worth choosing lower-alcohol versions or learning the alcohol content of your favourite brand to help you estimate how much you are drinking. There are websites that will calculate how many units there are in a glass of your favourite tipple (see page 237).

THE SIZE OF THE WINE GLASS

Just like burgers and choc bars, wine glass servings are getting bigger all the time. A lot of bars and pubs serve wine in larger glasses that may hold 250 ml (8 fl oz) of wine – this is as much as a third of a wine bottle. A glass of this size contains 3.3 units of alcohol, which is a woman's total alcohol allowance of the day! And a third of this glass would be equal to about one unit, which is the amount you're best to keep to if you're watching your weight. To make your wine go further, order a small glass of wine (125 ml/4 fl oz) instead and intersperse your alcohol drinks with low-calorie or diet drinks, or spritzers.

EVERYONE IS DIFFERENT

The guidelines are based on averages and no one person is the same as another. Factors such as height, weight, ethnicity and age will determine how much you can drink.

DON'T DRINK ON AN EMPTY STOMACH

This can make you drunk more quickly, but food in the stomach will help slow down the absorption of alcohol, especially if it's low-GI. Go for some breadsticks, crackers or unsalted nuts – remember, salty snacks will make you feel thirstier.

BINGE DRINKING

You may think you're not a binge drinker, but you might be surprised to know that if you down two large glasses of wine, you're officially considered a binge drinker – oops! Binge drinking is defined by the Office for National Statistics as eight or more units for a man and six or more units for a woman. This amounts to only two large glasses of wine for a woman.

꿈 Surround yourself with good company

DRINKING AND YOUR HEALTH

While there is some evidence to show that a glass of red wine may help reduce cardiovascular disease, other research shows that alcohol consumption may lead to numerous health problems. So, enjoy a drink but stick to your limits.

Nutritionists often call the calories in alcohol 'empty' calories. This is because you get very little in the way of nutrients such as vitamins and minerals. It is far better to get your calories from other foods that would be more beneficial to your health. For example, a small glass of wine (125 ml/4 fl oz) provides the same calories as one banana (90 g/3½ oz).

And there's a double whammy – drinking alcohol may also make you want to eat more. Alcohol stimulates the production of insulin, which leads to reduced blood sugar levels. This is what causes the pangs of hunger that you feel after a big night and makes you reach for more food.

Finally, alcohol is a diuretic so it makes you wee more. This leads to dehydration and that contributes to your hangover. Try to drink a glass of water between drinks to help your body to re-hydrate and prevent that hangover.

10 TOP TIPS

* Some drinks are much stronger than others, so switch from a strong drink, such as pure spirits, to a weak one, such as half a pint of lager of a lighter ABV.

* Decide on your units target before you go out – and stick to it.

* Top up your drinks with ice. This will dilute the drink and reduce the amount of alcohol you can get into the glass. Even a glass of white wine can be diluted with a few cubes of ice or try a spritzer if you don't like ice.

* Avoid top-ups as these make it hard to monitor how much you are drinking and you often drink more than you think.

* Take less money with you and leave your credit cards at home. This way you can determine how much you drink upfront.

* Tot up your units of alcohol while you're drinking. You will always be surprised and this can help you keep an eye on those units. Just as you benefit from eating consciously, try drinking consciously, too.

* Space out those drinks. Alternate glasses of water or soft drink with alcoholic drinks. Other options are a glass of mixer such as tonic. No one need know it is not a gin and tonic! This will help you stretch out your quota and prevent dehydration at the same time.

* Always try to eat when drinking as it helps to digest the alcohol more slowly. Eating something before you have a drink will also help.

* Sip, don't gulp.

* Try to give your body a break. Having at least two alcohol-free days every week will help your liver repair itself. You may even want to try an alcohol-free month!

Chat more, drink less

BEATING THE BOOZE

When we do things on auto-pilot, like going out on a Friday night for a long booze-up, we are less conscious of how much we're drinking. Being aware of what makes you drink, how much you drink and what you'll achieve if you cut down, can all be good motivation strategies. Instead of the drink having power over you, you'll begin to be truly in charge. Here are some suggestions to help you reduce the amount you drink.

BEFORE YOU START

✳ Write up a list of pros and cons. This is just two columns with one outlining the benefits for you of cutting down on drinking (e.g. you'll have more money for clothes) and the other listing the disadvantages of continuing to drink as much (e.g. weight gain). Keep this somewhere safe so you can refer to it at a later stage to remind yourself why you wanted to cut down.

✳ Make a plan. Work out what your strategy is before starting. This strategy will be personal to you and must be realistic. For example, you may want to limit yourself to two glasses of wine twice a week or you may prefer to make every second week an alcohol-free week. Think about when your plans may be sabotaged and come up with a remedy. Mark important milestones in your diary. Most importantly, make sure your strategy is realistic and achievable.

✳ Get your partner or friend to join in, and support each other.

RECORDS AND REWARDS

✳ Keep a diary. Write down every drink you have and revisit your diary weekly to monitor progress. Analysing your diary will point out where you may be having difficulties and help you work out some solutions.

✳ Drinking less means spending less. Estimate how much you spend each time you go out for drinks. Then calculate how much you spent each month on alcohol. Create a savings account or money pot that you can put all your savings into monthly.

✳ Reward yourself. Each time you reach an important milestone in your strategy, dip into your money pot and treat yourself to a trip to the theatre or a new accessory.

EIGHT ANTI-TEMPTATION TIPS

✳ Each time you get the urge to have a drink, distract yourself. Cravings may last less than five minutes and can be easily beaten by deep breathing, for example.

✳ Break some other habits. Associations between alcohol and some occasions can be very strong and the best way to tackle these may be to avoid those situations at first. For example, if you usually go out with colleagues for a drink after work try having lunch together in a café instead.

✳ Create some new routines. New activities such as dance classes may be a good distraction and can also boost your resolve.

✳ Understand what having another drink or drinking excessively, does for you. Whatever emotional need isn't being fulfilled, the answer isn't in the bottle! Find alternative, healthier ways of facing this head-on. For example, if it's boredom, use distractions such as a new interest. Perhaps find someone with the same interest, who will encourage you. Ask for the support you need to ensure that you succeed. A little of what you fancy really can do you good, just watch the balance!

✳ If you have limited yourself to your recommended daily units, enjoy and savour each sip, slowly. And when it's gone, it's gone!

✳ Think positively. Reducing your alcohol intake may not be easy but the benefits will become apparent after a few weeks. Don't use an excuse such as a crisis or good news to increase your alcohol intake.

✳ Treat yourself by using the money you've saved to buy yourself something special.

✳ Since alcoholic drinks tend to be high in calories, the more you drink the more calories you will be taking in. So less is definitely better.

🐌 *Relax more. Turn off the mobile!*

DRINKING DIARY

Keep a drinking diary for a week and make a note each time you have an alcoholic drink.

	Time of day	Where were you?	How much did you drink?
Day 1			
Day 2			
Day 3			
Day 4			
Day 5			
Day 6			
Day 7			

ANALYSING YOUR DRINKING DIARY

After a week, look at your drinking diary then answer these questions:

* In what sort of situations was I drinking more than I had intended to?
* Where did these situations occur?
* Who was I with?
* Did I have fun?
* Did I go through any guilt?
* Would it have been just as much fun if I hadn't overdone it?
* What have I learnt? What will I do differently next time when faced with similar situations?

Write down your answers/comments on the above questions as these will help you plan your own personal strategy.

YOUR PERSONAL STRATEGY

By answering the above questions, you may have identified situations where you are tempted to drink more. This knowledge will help you to plan your personal strategy for reducing your alcohol intake.

AND FINALLY...

* Make your wine go further by topping up your glass with mineral water or a diet lemonade.
* At the pub, make sure you're having standard pub measures rather than more generous servings. Make a spritzer with 25 ml (1 fl oz) of gin or vodka and add a calorie-free mixer.

✳ Choose a long slender glass rather than a short chunky one. It may trick your brain into thinking you're drinking more. Our eyes generally focus more on height than on volume so you may get more satisfaction drinking from a tall glass.

CHAPTER SIX:
GET GiP-FIT

Your age, weight, height and environment, what you eat, and how much you exercise all play a factor in determining your Basic Metabolic Rate (BMR). This is the very minimum amount of calories you need in a day in order to maintain whatever weight you are at and basically survive. So, if you are sitting idle, doing nothing all day, this is the number of calories you need to do that. In general, men have a higher BMR than women. And it may surprise you to know that a fatter person will generally have a higher (NOT lower) BMR than a thinner person. So you can't go using your metabolism as an excuse for being overweight any more!

When you restrict calories, you shed weight, but an extremely low-calorie diet is your metabolism's worst enemy. Your body needs a certain number of calories just to keep you alive – your BMR – plus a little more to support your level of activity. When you severely restrict calories your body thinks you are in starvation mode and it becomes very efficient at laying down fat stores – it also starts to use muscle mass for fuel because it's not getting enough energy from food.

❧ *Sit straight for healthier digestion*

Your body will consequently have relatively more fat than muscle, which means that your body needs even fewer calories to survive. If you plan on keeping to a strict low-calorie diet for life, this change in your metabolism may not be a problem but this would be virtually impossible, unnecessary and unhealthy in the long term. So, as soon as you go back to your normal eating habits, you gain the weight back – in the form of fat. Then it becomes even more difficult to lose the weight again because there is a lot more fat and a lot less muscle to help burn off that fat.

❧ Daily activity can reduce your 'real' age

Low-calorie eating triggers your body to think it's going through a famine so it saves vital energy by slowing down your metabolism. Even worse, your body learns to be more efficient at fat storage in case the famine happens again, so it can actually lead to future weight gain.

So how many calories should you cut down on to prevent your body from going into starvation mode and burning up lean muscle instead of fat? A 500-calorie-a-day deficit is the best way to safely and effectively lose weight long term – and this plan helps you to achieve just that, nice and slow and steady, helping your body to work with you and not against you.

CHOOSE EXERCISE YOU ENJOY AND BUILD IT INTO YOUR DAILY ROUTINE

There is an inextricable link between mind and body, and exercise releases endorphins (well-being chemicals). Thinking like an active person and including that as part of your identity, sends a useful message to your brain to act like that person. Remember, your actions are governed by your identity, who you believe yourself to be.

Just the recommended amount of physical activity, daily, makes a difference. For good health, it's recommended that you engage in five 30-minute sessions of moderate-intensity physical activity each week. That equates to 150 minutes a week. There is evidence to show that even if you split your activity into 10- or 15-minute chunks, this can give you the same benefits, provided you are working to moderate intensity. You should feel warm and slightly out of breath, but still able to hold a conversation. (And remember to check with your GP first if you're not used to exercising.)

> ❧ 'Acting on the advice of the authors, I decided
> to start by increasing my level of daily activity
> but in such a way so as I could effortlessly build
> it into my daily routine. After practising the
> visualisation techniques, which I found to be
> very powerful, I was able to see myself cycling to
> and from work at least four times a week.'

The Hot Body Plan, true to form, makes your life easier. Instead of having to do 30-minute workouts (unless you want to, of course) we suggest you have just two 10-minute bursts of physical activity every day. This is 140 minutes a week and we think that's good enough for you to make a start towards your new healthier lifestyle. More is obviously better, but whatever you do, build up to it gradually.

Choose your activity (the list overleaf will help you) and enjoy either two lots of 10–15-minute bursts (perhaps am and pm), or combine into a 20–30-minute workout.

How many reasons do you need to be convinced of the benefits of any kind of physical activity? Here are our reminders:

✳ Improves muscular strength
✳ Develops flexibility
✳ Helps prevent varicose veins
✳ Enhances posture
✳ Aids lower-back pain and strengthens the spine
✳ Helps to reduce anxiety, tension and stress
✳ Enhances self-esteem and confidence
✳ Helps prevent premature ageing
✳ Supports a balanced and healthy diet
✳ Helps to beat the blues
✳ Helps to keep up a healthy body image and good sex life
✳ Burns calories
✳ Reduces the risk of heart disease, osteoporosis and cancer

And much more!

CHOOSE YOUR DAILY ACTIVITY

✳ Brisk walking
✳ Cycling
✳ Jogging
✳ Dancing
✳ Running
✳ Swimming
✳ Marching on the spot
✳ Walking or running up and down the stairs
✳ Using the bottom stair as an 'aerobic stepper', using alternate feet to step up and down

The emphasis here is to love what you choose and choose what you love. A moderate, regular amount of exercise supports a regular, maintainable amount of weight- and inch-loss. Keep GiP-fit!

HOW TO LOSE ½ KG (1 LB) A WEEK – THE CALORIE CONNECTION

Your weight typically fluctuates every day. True weight change happens over a week or so, and to lose weight you need to be consistently taking in fewer calories than you are using up in your daily activities. Here's the maths: a pound of body fat contains 3500 calories (kcal), so to lose one pound in a week, you need to be eating:

3500 ÷ 7 = 500 kcal fewer each day.

If you think about it, this is a really simple way to steadily lose weight. If you could only find a way to cut down 500 calories each day, or use up 500 more calories by exercising, or a combination of both, your weight loss would just take care of itself.

❧ *Being active daily is your catalyst*

HOW TO BURN OFF 500 CALORIES

Choose five of these activities each day to use up 500 calories (remember, these figures are averages and people do vary):

Activity	Time (minutes)	Calories burnt
Skipping with a skipping rope	12	100
Gardening (digging)	15	100
Walking up and down the stairs	15	100
Walking briskly	20	100
Cycling at 16 kph (10 mph)	20	100
Cleaning windows	40	100
Hoovering energetically	40	100

Or choose two of these activities:

Activity	Time (minutes)	Calories burnt
High-impact aerobics	15	250
Jogging at 10 kph (6 mph)	25	250
Swimming at a moderate pace	30	250
Aqua aerobics	50	250
Dancing salsacise	50	250

Or choose to skip five 100-calorie snacks or two 250-calorie snacks to cut down your 500 calories:

Skip this...	Calories saved
1 large glass of wine	100
1 small café latte	100
1 chocolate-coated biscuit	100
1 medium jam doughnut	250
1 small flapjack	250
1 small chocolate bar	250

Or combine one or more activity with skipping a couple of snacks to end the day 500 calories short of your usual day's total. For example, you could aim for 12 minutes skipping, 10 minutes brisk walking and 15 minutes digging in the garden and forgo that jam doughnut. That's 500 calories. Vary the activities each day and make sure you always dodge at least one of your usual high-calorie treats. After one week this translates to ½ kg (1 lb) of weight lost. And if you use the GI advice in this Hot Body Plan, you will be satisfying your appetite and helping your overall health while you slim.

> ⁓ 'Mainly, my bike ride takes me along the
> shore beneath the cliffs. Some days, I watch and
> listen to the giant waves crashing, and other
> times, I'm in awe of the tranquility of the sea's
> calm. All the while, I'm consciously aware that I'm
> burning up the cals, thinking myself thin and
> every so often, pushing myself to add extra effort
> to the ride by increasing the time or going uphill.
> Oh yes, and some days are strictly for play only,
> like letting go of the handle bars and chuckling
> aloud as I very nearly come off, much to the
> delight of the passers-by!'

Also, to generally boost your energy expenditure try to integrate activity into your everyday life:

✳ Limit the time you spend sitting down watching TV and at the computer.
✳ At work, use the toilets on another floor of the building.
✳ Get off the bus early and walk some of the way home from work.

∗ Park at the edge of the car park and walk further to reach your destination.

∗ In the office, send work to a printer that is on the other side of the building so you have to walk a bit more.

∗ At work, instead of sending an email to someone who sits nearby, walk over to them.

∗ Use the local shops – and walk there and back or get on your bike.

∗ When shopping in a supermarket allow extra time and instead of working your way down the shop, go back and forth from one end to another to collect items.

∗ Use the garden as a place to exercise by digging up those beds, painting the fence and mowing the lawn to burn off some calories.

∗ Do an extra household job a week, such as washing the windows. Do this to music you enjoy, which will encourage you to move about.

∗ Join a local sports team or exercise class with a friend.

∗ If you have kids, take them to the park and join in a game of football or rounders.

∗ Go dancing with friends instead of to a pub or restaurant.

∗ Don't use the remote control for a TV, get up, walk to the TV and change channels or adjust the volume.

∗ Sign up for a hike or sponsored run/walk that involves training, so you have to do some sort of activity for a few months leading up to the event.

∗ When taking trains, take the long way round the station to other platforms to get connecting trains.

∗ For the days when you prefer the comfort of your own home, buy an exercise/fitness DVD – there are plenty to choose from – and join in!

&ac 'My husband and I started on the diet at the same time and we both lost 6 kg (13 lb) in 14 weeks. Both hubby and I tried it out and we progressed over the 14 weeks. On average I would say that I did two hours of exercise per week consisting of toning and aerobics. This diet made me very aware of the blood sugar levels rising slowly, prevention of diabetes, lower incidence of heart disease and improved levels of 'good' cholesterol. Despite going over the amounts allowed per week, I still managed to lose the weight. I have been very mindful of carbohydrates and am glad to say that I have kept most of my weight off.'

YOUR DAILY ACTIVITY CHART

CHART YOUR ACTIVITY PROGRESS

Use this chart to record how many of the 10-minute moderate-intensity activity sessions you're doing each day. Simply pencil in a tick every time, aiming for two ticks per day.

Day	Fitness burst 1	Fitness burst 2

And, to give you a tangible way of tracking your progress over time, fill in our Food and Exercise Log on pages 138–41.

BEAT THOSE BRAIN BLOCKS AND BUST THE BULGE!

You want to exercise, but sometimes it can seem like there are too many mental hurdles blocking your way. Here are some common excuses for not doing exercise and some great motivational pointers to show you how to beat those brain blocks. Borrow a Bulge Buster to enhance your sense of well-being.

'I'M IN SUCH BAD SHAPE, IT'S POINTLESS.'

Sometimes there is a sense of overwhelmingness that gets in the way of taking even that first small step. Just remember that the smallest of changes often makes the most significant difference as the cumulative effect kicks in. Remember, a journey of a thousand miles starts with one small step. Make up your mind to take that step today and before you know it, you'll begin to see the fruits of your labour paying off.

Bulge busters

Choose to make the changes that fit effortlessly into your current lifestyle.

∗ Get off public transport one stop earlier and walk the rest of the way. Create as many similar types of opportunities as you can.

∗ Put more oomph into everyday chores and without even leaving the house, know and feel those calories burning. For example: pretty much all household work; gardening and even pacing up and down while talking on the phone.

✳ Eating healthily and treating yourself to a dose of daily activity = looking fab and feeling great.

❧ Watch your posture, tuck that tummy in

'I CAN'T BE BOTHERED!'

Motivation is the key to success when it comes to achieving any goal in your life. Your mind needs to be constantly reminded of all the great benefits that will come when you succeed. Typically, the mind will look for the least painful and most effortless route to getting what it wants. Focus on the pleasure and on how great you'll feel.

Bulge busters

Make a list of all the benefits of going for it. Then bring it on!

✳ Get support from an exercise buddy. Work hard together and reward yourselves by playing hard, too! This includes a lot of laughs along the way.

✳ Surround yourself with the company of others who value their health and fitness. This will rub off on you, too.

✳ Choose a new interest or hobby that you'd love to try and sign up. It may be that you've been thinking about local jive or kick-boxing classes.

'GYM – SIN, NOT FOR ME!'

A routine trip to the gym is not everyone's cuppa, by any means. In fact, some find it downright boring. So, if this isn't for you, what is? You have so many options by simply making your daily life more active.

Bulge busters

✳ Just for fun, buy a pedometer to track how many steps you take in a day. Over a period of time, increase the number. When you're ready, set your own little challenge by brisk walking, then jogging and then running.

✳ Invent your own log book where you can keep track of all the small changes you are making. Aim for a new change every couple of days. For example, walking to your local supermarket, or store, or sandwich shop, daily.

'GETTING OFF THE COUCH – IT'S SUCH A DRAG!'

Even die-hard exercisers, on some days, would rather sink into the armchair and stay put. However, there's something to be said for giving yourself a pep talk, gritting your teeth and jumping to it!

Bulge busters

Giving it a go and getting out of the door is the first hurdle. Having got this far, remind yourself of the pain of not achieving and compare it to the sense of achievement you'll feel in 10 or 15 minutes' time.

✳ If it's a walk or a run that you're aiming for, say to yourself that you'll do a quick one. The chances are that you'll over-achieve and that will match your sense of satisfaction.

✳ On certain days, you can vary your choice of exercise by staying indoors and working out to an exercise DVD or dancing to your favourite CD tracks.

✳ Give yourself periodic rewards after x number of weeks. For example, a pedicure, manicure or a massage. It'll give you time to save your pennies, too.

'I JUST HAVEN'T GOT THE TIME!'

Never enough hours in a day, never enough days in a week and so it goes on. The funny thing is that whether you have 5 or 50 minutes, you'll still achieve what you set out to do when you're determined to do it. If you want something done well, give it to a busy person!

Bulge busters

Fail to plan and plan to fail. You probably already make a shopping list for the days or weeks ahead. Build a mini list or plan for your exercise for the same length of time and stick to it. The housework will still be there if you don't do it, but you can't buy back your exercise time!

* Make your daily activity plan such that it effortlessly fits in with your current lifestyle. This could mean walking the kids to school, which would be as great for them as it is for you. Or marching on the spot while you're cooking or waiting for the kettle to boil.
* You only need to schedule two 10-minute bursts. If you can manage more than this on most days, all well and good. Make sure it's something you enjoy, which boosts your sense of satisfaction. This way, you'll be even more motivated to carry on.

'I'VE GOT THE BLUES.'

One of the great reasons to make time for regular physical activity is that while you're exercising, the chances are that it'll keep your mind off any worries and woes that you may be carrying around. During exercise, the brain is releasing its so-called happy chemicals (endorphins), which provide an immediate lift, leaving you feeling upbeat and uplifted.

Bulge busters

* If for no other reason, prevention is better than cure! So, build in some daily activity knowing that it will help you stay uplifted.

* People who choose regular physical activity are less likely to be affected by the blues, through keeping motivated. Waking up to a feeling of optimism, ready to face the day ahead with a renewed sense of enthusiasm, is a great start to anyone's day.

Day of week	Time of day	Type of food and drink	Amount of food and drink
Monday			
Breakfast	e.g. 8 a.m.	e.g. bran-based cereal, semi-skimmed milk	e.g. 2 wheat biscuits, cereal bowl full of bran flakes
Snack			
Lunch			
Snack			
Dinner			
Tuesday			
Breakfast			
Snack			
Lunch			
Snack			
Dinner			
Wednesday			
Breakfast			
Snack			
Lunch			
Snack			
Dinner			

* Research suggests that optimists live longer than pessimists! So, prolong your life.

WEEKLY FOOD AND EXERCISE LOG

Use this diary to assess how you're doing. Making a note will give you feedback – see if there are any patterns in your behaviour and if any adjustments need to be made. You may want to make an enlarged photocopy.

Where	Your mood at the time	How did it make you feel afterwards?	Type and duration of activity
e.g. home, party, work	e.g. happy, sad, bored	e.g. energised	e.g. walking for 20 minutes

Day of week	Time of day	Type of food and drink	Amount of food and drink
Thursday			
Breakfast			
Snack			
Lunch			
Snack			
Dinner			
Friday			
Breakfast			
Snack			
Lunch			
Snack			
Dinner			
Saturday			
Breakfast			
Snack			
Lunch			
Snack			
Dinner			
Sunday			
Breakfast			
Snack			
Lunch			
Snack			
Dinner			

Where	Your mood at the time	How did it make you feel afterwards?	Type and duration of activity

AND FINALLY...

✳ The more energy you use in moving around, the faster your weight loss is likely to be. Exercise burns calories. Every time you move, you burn calories. So simply losing the TV remote control for a week can make you burn calories.

✳ Find your exercise prime time. Some people prefer to bounce out of bed and jog around the block before breakfast. Others prefer to go to the gym after work to relieve tension. You may prefer a brisk walk after dinner. Find your exercise prime time and enjoy the invigorating routine. It really does give you more get-up-and-go.

✳ Exercise can boost your muscle cells' sensitivity to the hormone insulin. This makes your body even more efficient at using up glucose and keeping your blood glucose levels steady.

✳ Are you someone who waits till you have a big pile of things to take upstairs and then go up? Why not carry up each item as you come across it so you can burn a few extra calories each time.

✳ Research suggests that watching TV is associated with childhood obesity. A Harvard study of 68,000 women showed that those who regularly watched two hours of TV daily were at a greater risk of developing obesity and diabetes. Check the TV listings and decide which one or two programmes you really must see. This will free up lots of time for more energetic or sociable activities.

CHAPTER SEVEN:
THE RECIPES

VICTORIOUS VEGGIE

MAGNIFICENT MEAT AND POULTRY

FUNKY FISH

DAZZLING DRESSINGS AND SAUCES

DESIRABLE DESSERTS

VICTORIOUS VEGGIE

CHUNKY HUMMUS

10 minutes • Serves 4

Chickpeas are a great source of protein and fibre, and the fact that they are also low-GI makes them a great food when you're watching your waistline. When you purée carbs, the GI does rise a little, so this chunkier version helps keep the GI low.

This recipe is quick and easy and much cheaper than bought hummus. It lasts in the fridge for a few days and is such a nutritious food that it makes a great replacement to higher fat fillings and dips. Enjoy it in pitta bread, in a wrap, as a dip or relish, as a spread, or with a salad.

1 tin (410 g) chickpeas, drained
5–6 tbsp lemon juice, or as desired
Good pinch of garlic salt or ½ tsp crushed garlic with a pinch of salt
1–2 tbsp freshly chopped basil leaves
1 tbsp fresh coriander leaves
50 g (2 oz) half-fat soft cheese
¼ tsp tahini paste or sesame seeds
Freshly ground black pepper
Paprika powder, optional

✳ Simply blitz all the ingredients together in a food processor or blender (not too smooth), adjust the seasoning, sprinkle with paprika (if using) and chill in the refrigerator.

What's good about me?

Soluble fibre from beans, lentils, chickpeas and other legumes can help to reduce blood cholesterol. Standard hummus has added oil. This version is just as creamy, but lower in fat and calories.

How can I make V V P C?

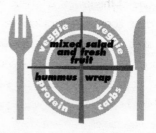

GUACAMOLE WITH BITE
5 minutes • Serves 2
Simple, substantial and scrumptious.

    1 ripe avocado
    1 tomato, finely chopped
    1 spring onion, sliced
    ½ pepper (red, yellow or orange), diced
    Generous pinch red chilli powder
    ¼ tsp crushed garlic
    2 tsp lemon juice

✳ Mash the avocado and mix it with the other ingredients.

What's good about me?
Packed with nutritious mono-unsaturated fats, avocados offer health in a jiffy. All you need to do is remove its packaging.

How can I make V V P C?

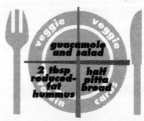

FASTA PASTA

20 minutes • Serves 2

Pasta is one of the lowest GI carbs so you can enjoy it regularly with a clear conscience, so long as you keep to the advised portion sizes (50 g/2 oz dried pasta per person). Fresh pasta only takes about four minutes to cook, and dried pasta around 10–12 minutes. The beauty of this recipe is that the vegetables are stir-fried while the pasta is boiling, so you save time. Choose your favourite vegetables – you already have the protein from the sweetcorn, the carb from the pasta, and veggie bits from the broccoli and tomatoes, so you get all the veggie veggie parts of your V V P C plate filled in one hit (for more on this, see page 63).

> 100 g (4 oz) pasta shapes (choose whichever you like)
> 1 tsp olive oil
> 2 onions, sliced
> 1 tsp crushed garlic
> 300 g (11 oz) frozen or fresh broccoli florets
> 325 g tin sweetcorn, drained
> 150 ml (5 fl oz) virtually fat-free fromage frais
> 2 tbsp freshly chopped parsley
> Good pinch dried herbs of your choice
> 3 tomatoes, cut into wedges

* Boil the pasta in a pan of lightly salted water until just cooked.
* Meanwhile, heat a non-stick pan and add the olive oil. Stir-fry the onions and garlic in the hot oil for a couple of minutes.
* Add the broccoli and allow to cook till just tender, stirring frequently.
* Throw in all the other ingredients with the drained cooked pasta and heat thoroughly.

What's good about me?

The flexibility of this dish allows you to chuck in any leftovers, including chicken, fish or vegetables so that you can create a substantial meal in minutes. You get at least two portions of vegetables from just one serving.

How can I make V V P C?

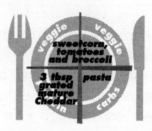

- -

HONEYED MANGE TOUT

10 minutes • Serves 2

If steamed or boiled vegetables don't do it for you, you can always try different methods of flavouring and cooking. This recipe stir-fries fresh mange tout in a small amount of honey, which adds a little sweetness and also helps to caramelise the peas. Each serving has only half a teaspoon of honey, which really isn't worth worrying about.

> 10 sprays of spray oil
> 150 g (5 oz) mange tout
> 1 tsp herbes de Provence
> Salt and pepper
> 1 tsp honey

* Heat a non-stick pan and add 10 sprays of oil.
* Stir-fry the mange tout with the herbs and seasoning until cooked, about 8–10 minutes.
* Stir in the honey near the end of cooking and allow to caramelise on a high heat.

What's good about me?

Different coloured vegetables offer you a different range of nutrients. Mange tout are a good source of beta-carotene, which is converted into vitamin A in the body.

ASPARAGUS ANTICIPATION

10 minutes • Serves 2

Asparagus is sometimes called 'the king of spring vegetables'. It was once considered a luxury, but now is more affordable and this speedy recipe makes a delicious accompaniment to any meat or fish.

> 10 sprays of spray oil
> 250 g (9 oz) fresh asparagus spears
> 1–2 tbsp balsamic vinegar
> Freshly ground black pepper
> ½ red onion, finely chopped (optional)

* Heat 10 sprays of oil in a non-stick pan.
* Add the asparagus and stir-fry for 5–7 minutes, turning, until just tender.
* Serve immediately, drizzled with the balsamic vinegar, seasoned, and scattered with crisp red onion.

What's good about me?

Asparagus is really versatile. You can steam, boil, griddle, roast, barbecue or stir-fry it as above.

VEGGIE BULGUR WHEAT

20 minutes • Serves 2

This is cracked wheat, not commonly used in British cooking. It is so fantastically low in GI, however, that it is really worth experimenting with.

> 400 ml (14 fl oz) made-up vegetable stock, boiled
> 100 g (4 oz) bulgur wheat
> Generous pinch of dried mixed herbs
> Pinch of salt
> ½ red pepper, diced
> ½ yellow pepper, diced
> Handful of fresh coriander leaves, roughly chopped
> 2 tomatoes, chopped
> 2 courgettes, sliced
> ½ tsp red chilli powder (optional)
> Coarse black pepper
> 1–2 tbsp lemon juice

✳ Heat the stock and add all the other ingredients except the lemon juice. Stir well and cook in a covered saucepan for 10–12 minutes, until the water is absorbed.

✳ Mix well; squeeze in the lemon juice and serve hot or cold.

What's good about me?

Bulgur wheat has a lower GI than even basmati rice, and is much lower than potatoes. Choose it as an accompaniment often. You can flavour it as you like. If you fancy this as a main vegetarian meal, add the protein part using a pot of low-fat natural yoghurt or a raita (see page 171), or simply throw in some crushed walnuts or cubed feta cheese.

CABBAGE WITH FENNEL SEEDS

10 minutes • Serves 4

If thinking of cabbage conjures up images of soggy cabbage at school dinners, then try this version, which boasts lightly cooked white cabbage with the unusual taste of fennel seeds. This dish works well with grated carrots and shredded savoy cabbage too – use a combination of equal amounts of each.

450 g (1 lb) white cabbage, sliced
1 tsp olive oil
2 tbsp fennel seeds
Salt and coarsely ground black pepper
Pinch of cayenne pepper

* Steam the cabbage in a covered pan until just cooked. Drain.
* Heat the oil. Add the fennel seeds and let them pop for a few seconds. Then add the cabbage and stir-fry, season, sprinkle on some cayenne pepper and serve.

What's good about me?

Fibre, crunch and anti-oxidants, especially if you steam the cabbage in the minimum of water.

THAI BABY CORN AND MANGE TOUT WITH CRUSHED PEANUTS
10–15 minutes • Serves 4

200 g (7 oz) fresh baby corn
1 tsp sesame oil
175 g (6 oz) mange tout
6 spring onions, roots removed and chopped diagonally
   (approximately 2 cm/¾ in long)
2 tsp Thai fish sauce
Handful of basil leaves, torn
75 g (3 oz) chopped peanuts
2 tbsp chopped coriander leaves

✳ Part-cook the baby corn by heating in the microwave in water for 3 minutes on High (or simmer for the same time in a saucepan).

✳ Drain and then cut each corn cob in half lengthways.

✳ Heat a wok to a high temperature then add the sesame oil.

✳ Add the mange tout, spring onions, fish sauce, basil and baby corn pieces and continue to stir-fry on a high heat for 3 minutes.

✳ Sprinkle with the nuts and coriander, and serve.

What's good about me?
Peanuts are certainly high in fat, but it's the healthy mono-saturated type. Nuts also have a low glycaemic index so they can actually help keep your blood glucose levels steady. Sprinkle them into foods in this way so that you add valuable nutrients – a handful a day is perfectly acceptable as part of a healthy diet.

How can I make V V P C?

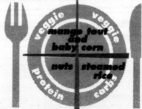

MINTED PEAS
5 minutes • Serves 2

Few sprays of spray oil
225 g (8 oz) frozen peas
1 tsp mint sauce
Generous pinch of dried mixed herbs
A little salt

✳ Spray some oil onto a microwavable dish and add the peas with 1–2 tbsp of water.

✳ Stir in the other ingredients and cook in the microwave for about 4 minutes, turning halfway through cooking. Check they are tender, adjust seasoning and cook a little further if required.

What's good about me?
Peas are a good source of potassium, helping to keep your blood pressure low.

CREAMY ASPARAGUS SOUP
10 minutes • Serves 2

1 tsp rapeseed oil
1 onion, chopped
½ tsp crushed garlic
600 ml (1 pint) skimmed milk
Generous pinch of dried mixed herbs
1 vegetable stock cube
1 heaped tsp cornflour
250 g (9 oz) asparagus, chopped
Salt and pepper

To serve
2 slices granary bread
1 tbsp freshly chopped dill

✳ Heat the oil in a non-stick pan and fry the onion and garlic to soften.

✳ Add the milk, herbs and stock cube and warm through over a low heat – don't cover the pan as the milk will boil over.

✳ Mix the cornflour with a little cold water, add this to the pan and stir until boiling and thickened.

✳ Stir in the asparagus and season to taste.

✳ Cut the bread into crouton-sized pieces, and toast on both sides under a medium grill till brown.

✳ Serve the soup hot, topped with fresh dill and croutons.

What's good about me?
This dish is low in fat because it's made from skimmed milk, and it gives you protein and calcium.

CHINESE NOODLE AND BABY CORN SOUP
5 minutes • Serves 2

A quick, easy and satisfying soup made from a packet of instant noodles.

> 108 g packet instant noodles
> 1 tin (200 g) baby sweetcorn
> Few drops sesame oil
> 3 spring onions, sliced diagonally

* Simply throw everything into a pot and cook as suggested on the noodle packet, normally for about 3 minutes.

What's good about me?
Noodles are a tasty low-GI food.

CELERY BOATS
5 minutes • Serves 1

> 1 tbsp ricotta cheese
> Good pinch dried basil
> Few chives, snipped
> 1 stick celery, cut into 8-cm (3-in) sticks
> Black pepper, to taste
> Paprika, to taste

* Mix the cheese with the basil and chives.
* Fill the celery boats and season with black pepper and paprika.

What's good about me?
Low calories, low saturated fat, high taste!

FRUITY BULGUR WITH CASHEW NUTS

15 minutes • Serves 4

You really need to try bulgur wheat – it's so versatile, and adding turmeric gives it a vibrant colour, great for kids too. You can use any fruit or nuts you like but I find dried apricots with cashews work well.

> 800 ml (1¼ pints) of made-up vegetable stock, boiled
> 200 g (7 oz) bulgur wheat
> Pinch ground turmeric
> Generous handful of dried apricots (around 15), chopped
> Juice of 1 orange
> 50 g (2 oz) cashew nuts (about 40 nuts)

* Simply mix all the ingredients together in a non-stick pan, cover and cook for about 12–15 minutes over a medium heat.

What's good about me?

One serving gives you your carbs, protein and one fruit portion.

MAGNIFICENT MEAT AND POULTRY

TERIYAKI CHICKEN STRIPPERS
10 minutes • Serves 2
You can use chicken, fish or even red meat for this speedy dish. Serve it either on its own, with a dip or as a starter. Alternatively, it is delicious served in a tortilla wrap with crunchy fresh salad vegetables.

> *2 chicken breasts, skin removed, cut into strips*
> *2 tbsp teriyaki sauce*
> *½ tsp crushed garlic*
> *Black pepper or red chilli powder, as desired*
> *1 tsp olive or rapeseed oil*
> *Fresh lime or lemon wedges, to serve*

* Marinate the chicken in the sauce, garlic and seasoning.
* Heat the oil in a large non-stick frying pan or wok. Stir-fry the flavoured chicken until cooked and serve immediately with the lime or lemon wedges.

What's good about me?
Chicken breast is low in fat and rich in protein – protein foods help to fill you up.

SAUCY CHOPS
15 minutes • Serves 2

You can use lamb or pork chops for this finger-licking dish – great for grilling, barbecuing or oven-baking. If you can, marinate the chops for a few hours as this will allow the flavours to really penetrate the meat. The easiest way to cook them is in an oven-proof dish covered in foil. They will bake gently, absorbing all the flavours yet still staying moist. Uncover the foil for about 5 minutes before serving so that the chops are lightly browned. The chops are cooked in a flavoured yoghurt sauce. If you prefer to serve some of the sauce on the side, then simply use less in the marinade.

> *4 lean lamb or pork chops*
> *300 ml (10 fl oz) low-fat natural yoghurt*
> *1 tsp crushed garlic*
> *1 tsp crushed ginger*
> *½ tsp dried rosemary*
> *½ tsp mint sauce (use more if you like it really minty)*

✳ Marinate the chops in all the other ingredients.

✳ Cook either under the grill, on a barbecue or covered in foil in a moderate oven until the juices run clear. Serve immediately.

What's good about me?
Lean red meat is a good source of iron, zinc and vitamin B12. Iron and zinc are great for helping you deal with fatigue.

PORK STEAKS WITH CREAMY MUSTARD SAUCE

20 minutes • Serves 4

Pork steaks are now much leaner and consequently lower in fat, so are an ideal meat to choose when trying to be health conscious. They are enhanced by the taste of mustard to make a delicious and convenient dish.

> Few sprays of spray oil
> 4 lean pork steaks (approximately 120 g/4½ oz each), trimmed of any fat
> 1 medium onion, finely chopped
> 150 ml (5 fl oz) chicken stock, hot
> 175 g (6 oz) low-fat natural yoghurt
> 1 dessertspoon whole grain mustard

* Heat a heavy-based frying pan or griddle, add the spray oil and pan-fry the pork steaks for 10 minutes.
* Remove from the pan and keep hot ready for serving.
* Add the onion to the residues in the frying pan, and cook until soft. Add the hot stock and cook for another 5 minutes.
* Remove from the heat and stir in the yoghurt and mustard. Gently reheat, stirring continuously and serve poured over the pork steaks.

What's good about me?

The sauce may be creamy, but there isn't an ounce of cream in sight!

SCOTCH EGGS

30 minutes, plus 20 minutes' cooking • Serves 4

These do take a bit of time, but are well worth the effort.

It's a lot easier if you have a mini food processor or grinder for the onion, chickpeas and the All Bran. However if you don't, simply grate the onion and use breadcrumbs (or drench a slice of granary bread under a tap, squeeze out the excess water and add this to the turkey mixture). You can crush the All Bran in a polythene bag using a rolling pin.

> 4 eggs
> 250 g (9 oz) minced turkey
> I onion, grated
> ¼ tin (100 g) chickpeas, puréed or I slice granary bread,
>   made into breadcrumbs
> I tsp crushed garlic
> 3 tbsp Worcestershire sauce
> ½ tsp mixed dried herbs
> ½–I tsp salt
> Coarse black pepper
> I egg, beaten
> 6 tbsp All Bran, crushed or ground
> Few sprays of spray oil

* Preheat the oven to 200°C/400°F/gas 6 and line a baking tray with foil.
* Hard-boil the eggs, cool and remove the shells.
* Meanwhile, mix together the turkey, onion, chickpeas (or breadcrumbs), garlic, Worcestershire sauce, mixed herbs, seasoning and beaten egg.
* Coat each egg with a quarter of the turkey mixture and then roll the Scotch eggs in the ground-up All Bran.

* Spray the baking tray with spray oil and place the made-up Scotch eggs on the tray, spraying some more oil over the top. Bake in the oven for 15–20 minutes.

What's good about me?

Anyone watching their weight knows that standard Scotch eggs would be out of bounds, particularly because they are high in saturated fat and because of the salty sausage meat. This recipe in comparison is far lower in fat and salt, and you even get some fibre from the All Bran!

LAMB CUTLETS WITH TOMATO AND MINT SAUCE

20 minutes • Serves 4

A refreshing and light sauce that combines well with the heaviness of lamb. This dish is ideal served with new potatoes and cauliflower.

4 lamb escalopes (approximately 100 g/4 oz each)
700 g (1½ lb) cherry tomatoes, halved
10 leaves of fresh mint (or 1 tsp mint sauce)
1 tsp sugar
Salt and freshly milled black pepper

* In a shallow, open pan, place the tomato halves with 2 tablespoons of water and the mint leaves, and simmer for 10 minutes until soft.
* Add the sugar (and mint sauce if using) and then liquidise.
* Season and reheat.
* Meanwhile grill the lamb cutlets on both sides under a medium heat until the juices run clear (5–10 minutes) and serve with the sauce.

FUNKY FISH

10-MINUTE TROUT WITH EXOTIC SEEDS

10 minutes • Serves 2

This dish is an unusual combination of delicate fish and flavour-some whole seeds. You can buy the onion and coriander seeds in most supermarkets, and especially in Asian grocery stores. The fish cooks very quickly, so make sure you have all your accompaniments ready. It goes well with *Honeyed Mange Tout* (see page 148).

> *15–20 sprays of spray oil*
> *½ tsp onion seeds*
> *2 fillets fresh trout*
> *½ tsp whole coriander seeds*
> *Salt and pepper*
> *3 tbsp lemon juice or a combination of lemon juice and white wine*

* Heat a non-stick frying pan over a medium heat and spray with 15–20 sprays of oil.

* Once the oil is heated, lower the heat, add the seeds and allow them to cook for a few seconds in the oil.

* Season the trout and place the fillets, skin side down, on top of the seeds. Allow to cook for about four minutes, and then turn the fish over.

* Add some of the lemon juice (or white wine) and cook the other side of the fish for around 3–4 minutes, depending on the thickness of the fillets. Drizzle the remaining lemon juice (or white wine) over the fish, and serve, skin side down. Spoon any remaining seeds on to the fish.

What's good about me?

Trout is a rich source of omega-3 fats, known to be heart-protective. There is also some research to show that the omega-3 oils may help improve concentration and memory.

- -

TIGER PRAWNS WITH CREAMY DIPPING SAUCE

5 minutes • Serves 2

Tiger prawns make a luscious addition to any dinner party. However, why save them only for special occasions? They are so quick to cook and versatile that it really is worth experimenting a little. You can either serve these prawns with the dipping sauce, or stuff them into a pitta bread or wrap. Alternatively serve them on toast or with salad. They are also fab with noodles.

I tsp olive oil
250 g (9 oz) cooked tiger prawns
½ tsp crushed garlic
I tbsp white wine or lemon juice
Coarse black pepper

For the sauce

50 g (2 oz) virtually fat-free fromage frais
I tsp coarse grain mustard or ¼ tsp Dijon mustard
¼–½ tsp mint sauce

* Heat the oil in a non-stick frying pan or wok. Add the prawns with the flavourings and stir-fry for 3–4 minutes.
* Meanwhile, prepare the sauce by mixing together the sauce ingredients, adding seasoning if necessary.

POSH FISH FINGERS WITH TARTARE SAUCE

15 minutes • Serves 2

With this recipe, you can be sure that the only thing in your fish fingers is real fish. Also, these strips of cod are dipped in fresh orange juice and herbs before being lightly fried in olive oil. The beauty of home-cooked food as opposed to processed food is the natural shapes and textures, so enjoy the unevenness of these fish fingers. You can use either fresh or frozen cod. If using frozen, defrost the cod fillets for about an hour only, since if they are still slightly frozen, it will be easier to make sharp, straight cuts through each fillet.

2 cod fillets, fresh or frozen
¼–½ tsp dried mixed herbs
1 tbsp finely chopped fresh parsley
Salt and pepper
2–3 tbsp orange juice
Orange breadcrumbs
Fresh lemon, cut into wedges

For the sauce

100 ml (4 fl oz) low-fat Greek style yoghurt or virtually fat-
free fromage frais
1 heaped tbsp capers, chopped
1 spring onion, sliced (optional)
Freshly ground black pepper

✳ Preheat the grill and line the grill pan with foil, drizzled with some oil.

✳ Cut the cod fillets into thin strips. Season them with the herbs and seasoning.

✳ Pour the orange juice into a soup plate and sprinkle a generous amount of orange breadcrumbs onto a dinner plate.

* Dip the strips of cod first into the orange juice and then coat each strip with the breadcrumbs.
* Gently place the fish fingers onto the grill pan and drizzle or spray a little more oil on top. Cook under a medium grill for 5 minutes on each side or until fully cooked.
* Meanwhile, mix together the ingredients for the tartare sauce.
* Serve the cooked fish immediately with the sauce and fresh lemon wedges.

What's good about me?

Real cod means the food is as close to its natural state as possible, not processed.

TUNA AND SWEETCORN BASKETS
20 minutes, plus 15 minutes' cooking • Makes 10

A stunning yet healthy party piece. You will have some bread crusts left over – don't be tempted to nibble on them, just keep them aside for breadcrumbs or croutons for another day.

Few sprays of spray oil
10 slices granary bread
250 g (9 oz) ricotta cheese
150 g (5 oz) sweetcorn
185 g tinned tuna in brine, drained
2 tsp mixed herbs
2 tsp crushed garlic
Seasoning to taste
3 tbsp chopped fresh coriander leaves, optional
Sweet chilli sauce

* Preheat the oven to 200°C/400°F/gas 6. Spray a muffin tray or individual foil pastry cases with spray oil.

✳ Cut the bread into large circles – they should fit the base and part of the sides of the muffin or pastry cases.

✳ Line the cases with the bread circles and save the crusts for the basket handles.

✳ Mix the ricotta cheese with the sweetcorn, tuna, mixed herbs and garlic, and season to taste.

✳ Fill the bread cases with 1 heaped tablespoon of the tuna mixture. You should have enough mixture to fill 10 cases.

✳ Cut the crusts so that they are about the right length to be pushed into the tuna mixture and standup like a handle.

✳ Bake until the bread is toasted, around 15 minutes. Serve with a drizzling of sweet chilli sauce.

What's good about me?

This sort of dish would generally be made with pastry, but here you're using low-GI and lower-calorie bread with low-fat soft cheese.

DAZZLING DRESSINGS AND SAUCES

CORIANDER AND MINT CHUTNEY
5 minutes • Serves 4–6

A speedy accompaniment that dresses up any meal or party table. You can either use roughly chopped ingredients that add crunch, or you can mix this all together in a mini food processor.

> *25 g (1 oz) fresh coriander leaves and stems, chopped*
> *2 spring onions, sliced*
> *15 g (½ oz) fresh mint leaves, chopped*
> *¼ tsp crushed garlic*
> *Lemon juice, to taste*
> *Salt and pepper*

✳ Simply mix all the ingredients together or blitz in the food processor. Add lemon juice and seasoning to taste.

What's good about me?
No fat, no GiPs, no calories, lots of taste.

BALSAMIC AND HONEY DRESSING
5 minutes • Serves 2

> 1 tbsp balsamic vinegar
> ¼–½ tsp mustard
> 1 tsp honey
> Pinch dried oregano

✳ Simply mix the ingredients in a screw top jar, put the lid on and give it a shake! Drizzle over your favourite salads.

What's good about me?
Sometimes you need a flavour kick to help you eat the salads, so this one comes up trumps when you want flavour, not fat.

MINTY MOMENTS
5 minutes • Serves 2

> 2 tsp mint sauce
> 2 tsp ketchup
> 2 tbsp water
> ½ –1 tsp red chilli powder, as desired

✳ Just mix together the ingredients, adjust to taste and serve with lamb dishes or salads.

What's good about me?
This sauce helps when your dinner needs a hasty makeover.

SHAI'S SALSA

5 minutes • Serves 4

Thanks to our dear friend Shairoz for this tangy, tasty recipe.

1 red pepper, roughly chopped
1 green pepper, roughly chopped
Handful of fresh coriander leaves
Small red onion, roughly chopped
3 tomatoes, roughly chopped
1–2 green chillies, roughly chopped
Pinch of salt
Pinch of sugar
2 tbsp lemon juice
1 tsp crushed garlic or 1 garlic clove

* Blitz all of the ingredients together in a food processor and devour.

What's good about me?

Have you seen those colours? Red and green galore provide a nice variety of nutrients. The acidic lemon juice will help lower the GI of other foods you eat with this salsa, a double whammy!

GARLIC SAUCE
5 minutes • Serves 2–3

> 150 ml (5 fl oz) low-fat natural yoghurt
> 1–2 tsp crushed garlic
> 2 tbsp finely chopped coriander leaves
> Coarse black pepper

✳ Just mix together the ingredients and adjust to taste. This goes well with kebabs and salad.

What's good about me?
No mayonnaise or oil, just low-fat yoghurt, herbs and garlic – taste on a plate!

CUCUMBER RAITA DIP

5 minutes • Serves 4

A cooling accompaniment that gives you one of your three-a-day calcium portions.

> 500 ml (18 fl oz) low-fat natural yoghurt
> ½ tsp cumin seeds
> Ground black pepper
> ½ tsp dried mint
> 3 tbsp finely chopped coriander leaves
> ⅓ of a cucumber, finely diced

✳ Mix together all the ingredients except the cucumber, and chill in the refrigerator till you are ready to serve. Stir in the cucumber just before serving.

What's good about me?

You can use this as one of your protein servings on V V P C – so it could team up well with a steamed vegetable rice (where you have two veggies and one carb from the rice).

REALLY USEFUL CURRY BASE
10 minutes • Serves 2

This is a great sauce to use as a base for any curry. It only takes about 10 minutes to prepare and you just need to add in your favourite tin of beans, chunks of chicken breast, prawns, whatever you like to make it into a delicious homemade Indian treat. Serve up with some steamed basmati rice and cooling natural yoghurt.

> 1 tsp rapeseed oil
> 1 tsp onion seeds
> ½ tsp black mustard seeds
> 1 tsp cumin seeds
> 200 g (7 oz) tinned chopped tomatoes
> 1–2 tsp crushed garlic
> 1 tsp crushed ginger
> 1–2 green chillies, chopped
> ¼ tsp ground turmeric
> 1 tsp ground coriander seeds

✳ Heat the oil in a non-stick pan over a low heat.

✳ Add all the seeds and allow to pop for only a few seconds before adding the tomatoes. Cover immediately to lock in the aroma. Stir well and cook for about 3–4 minutes until the tomatoes are well blended.

✳ Stir in the other ingredients, cover and simmer for a few minutes.

✳ Add your beans, meat or fish, or cool in the refrigerator for later use.

What's good about me?
Tinned tomatoes are packed with lycopene, a powerful anti-oxidant and you get one of your five a day just from the sauce!

UNIVERSAL PASTA SAUCE

15 minutes • Serves 4

Use this as a base for any pasta.

> 20 sprays of spray oil or 1 tsp rapeseed or olive oil
> 2 cloves garlic, crushed
> 1 onion, finely chopped
> 1 green pepper, diced
> 255 g (9 oz) tinned chopped tomatoes
> 1½ tsp dried oregano
> Salt and coarsely ground black pepper

* Heat the oil in a large non-stick pan. Add the garlic, onion and green pepper and fry until the onions are light brown (3–5 minutes).
* Pour in the tomatoes. Stir-fry until the tomatoes become soft and mushy (4–5 minutes). Add a little hot water if the mixture begins to stick to the bottom.
* Stir in the oregano and season to taste.

What's good about me?

A low-fat, flavoursome sauce packed with goodness.

DESIRABLE DESSERTS

RED FRUIT COMPOTE
5 minutes • Serves 4

Red fruit compote is an interesting variation on a traditional fruit salad. If desired you could leave the alcohol out all together or use 1 tablespoon of Cointreau instead of the wine.

> 150 g (5 oz) strawberries, hulled and cut into bite-sized pieces
> 100 g (4 oz) cherries, stoned
> 100 g (4 oz) raspberries
> 100 g (4 oz) blackberries
> 2–3 tbsp dry white wine, sparkling if possible
> 1 tbsp icing sugar
> Fresh mint sprigs

✳ Wash all the fruit and make sure it has been cut into bite-sized pieces.

✳ Place in a large serving bowl and pour over the wine. Sprinkle with icing sugar and leave in a cold place to chill.

✳ Mix once before serving and decorate with fresh mint.

What's good about me?
Berries are a rich source of fibre and vitamin C, as well as antioxidants that can help protect against heart disease.

MELON AND RASPBERRY WITH MINT
10 minutes • Serves 4

Impress your guests by using a melon baller and serving them in a melon shell. For extra wow factor, mix a variety of melon types, such as pink watermelon, pale honeydew and bright orange cantaloupe.

> 1 galia melon
> 250 g (9 oz) fresh raspberries, washed and hulls removed
> 3 sprigs of fresh mint (plus 8 mint leaves for garnish)
> 200 ml (7 fl oz) dry white wine, chilled

✳ Cut the melon into bite-sized pieces and discard the skin. Put in a bowl with the raspberries and bruised mint sprigs.

✳ Pour over the chilled wine and chill further for 5 minutes.

✳ Remove the bruised mint and serve the melon in individual glass dishes garnished with mint leaves.

What's good about me?
Refreshing and nourishing – the orange-coloured melons, such as cantaloupe, have beta-carotene.

WARM BANANAS WITH ORANGE
10 minutes • Serves 2

Fed up with fruit served the same old way? Then try this dish of warm, softened bananas.

> *5 sprays of spray oil*
> *1 banana, sliced diagonally*
> *3 tbsp orange juice*
> *Sprinkling of sesame seeds*

✳ Heat a non-stick frying pan and add 5 sprays of oil.
✳ Add the banana and sauté for a couple of minutes, adding the orange juice to prevent sticking.
✳ Serve immediately with a light sprinkling of sesame seeds.

What's good about me?

Choose green-tipped bananas since they are likely to have a lower-GI than ripe ones.

LYCHEES WITH PISTACHIO
5 minutes • Serves 2

> *1 tin (425 g) lychees, drained*
> *Pistachio nuts (1 for each lychee)*
> *1 tbsp sesame seeds*

* Stuff the inside of each lychee with one pistachio, leaving a bit of the nut exposed.
* Lightly toast the sesame seeds in a frying pan or under a grill. Be careful as they burn easily.
* Roll the stuffed lychees in the sesame seeds.

What's good about me?
Even tinned fruit counts towards your five a day – just make sure you drain the fruit well and go for types tinned in water or natural juice if you can.

GRILLED ORANGES
5 minutes • Serves 1

> *1 orange, halved*
> *1 tsp sugar*

* Preheat the grill to medium.
* Sprinkle the sugar on top of the orange halves and grill till browned.

What's good about me?
A new way to have your daily dose of vitamin C.

AND FINALLY...

✳ The recipes in this book can be conjured up in around 20 minutes. Remember to use shortcuts such as frozen, pre-cut or tinned vegetables, crushed garlic and dried herbs to keep it simple and speedy.

✳ When cooking, it's often very easy to get tempted to taste your creation. Put some raw vegetables on a plate instead, so that you can still nibble while you cook.

✳ If you need to fry foods, try spraying oil on a non-stick pan. Cook using a few sprays of spray oil rather than pouring oil from a bottle. Use a bought version or simply buy a spray bottle from a kitchenware store and pour in your favourite oil (we recommend rapeseed or olive oil), then use this in cooking. A few sprays will still mean you are using less than if you were pouring or using a tablespoon.

✳ Select lean cuts of meat and trim off visible fat. Try to cook meat without adding fat, by grilling, roasting and braising. Avoid using the juices from roast meat for gravy. Meat can stay moist if you use other liquid flavourings like stock, or lower-fat Greek yoghurt (lovely with poultry), and keep the lid on so you don't lose too much moisture.

✳ Pulses such as beans, sweetcorn, peas and lentils are generally low in calories and help to fill you up. Choose them often – if possible once a day.

✳ Eggs can be poached, boiled or scrambled instead of fried.

✳ Remember Mediterranean eating is healthy – garlic, fruit and veg, fish, nuts, beans and lentils are all foods we recommend in the Hot Body Plan.

✳ Choose foods that are low in salt, and go easy on added salt. Too much salt can make some people more prone to high blood pressure and we eat more than twice the salt we need.

CHAPTER EIGHT: TIME TO PARTY!

FEELIN' HOT, HOT, HOT!

It's time to party. You are the party! Be it on the beach or elsewhere. By now, you will be starting to feel great about yourself. The following exercise will ensure that you build on this feeling so that your presence and aura of confidence walks into a room even before your physical body! Remember, your body is a temple, but sometimes it's a nightclub and that's fine, too! Your preparation will pay off big time and with our great food and alcohol guide, you'll be in fine mental shape to follow it through without that need for overindulgence.

THE RING OF CONFIDENCE

✳ Find a quiet spot in- or outdoors. Imagine a magical and instant 'Ring of Confidence' a few steps in front of you. Make this picture bold, bright and colourful. When you can see this clearly in your mind's eye, step into it, and begin to feel an immediate and powerful surge of inner confidence.

✳ Take a few slow, deep breaths. On each breath, imagine you are pulling confidence up through the soles of your feet.

Allow this energy to make its way up your legs, abdomen, torso, into your head and out through the crown, so that it engulfs your whole body.

✳ Pay attention to the instant changes to your facial expression and as you sense this growth in confidence, notice how much straighter and taller you've become, literally growing in stature. Improve your posture even more by pulling in your tummy muscles, with your shoulders back, chest back and head held high. This will add to your air of confidence.

✳ Now see yourself at a party, on the beach or elsewhere. See how fantastic you look in the little black number, or equivalent, slim and trim. Your efforts have paid off. Notice the people around you and how they are drawn to you. Notice your positive self-talk and the way in which you are congratulating yourself. Others will be offering you their encouraging comments, too. Notice how GREAT you feel.

✳ At this point, you can find a personal 'trigger' that will allow you to access this feeling any time you want. Your 'trigger' can be a gesture you make, for example, punching the air, or an image or a sound, like an upbeat piece of music in your head, or a resounding Yesssssss! Alternatively, press your thumb and first finger together on one hand, or press a knuckle or an ear lobe. Anything that you choose, that will activate your instant personal trigger, so that you can recreate this positive feeling, anywhere, any time!

✳ Step out of the ring and back in, several more times until your feeling of confidence is automatically triggered, instantly.

Now that you are able to reach this peak state at will, you are ready to party the night or day away! You look your best, sound your best and feel your best.

THE PARTY

No need for you to be a party pooper, with our GI Hot Body tips for letting your hair down, you will be able to indulge and enjoy…

SUMPTUOUS PARTY SWAPS

Enjoy this…	*Because you don't need this…*
Bean salads	Cheesy salads, such as Caesar salad
Bits on cocktail sticks: olives, pickled onions, gherkins, cherry tomatoes	Bits on cocktail sticks: cheese
Bits on skewers: grilled kebabs, chicken souvlaki, fish, peppers, onion, tomatoes, mushrooms	Fried bits: breaded mushrooms, veg tempura, onion bhajis, samosas, spring rolls
Chicken without the skin (try recipe for Teriyaki Chicken Strippers)	Fried chicken drumsticks with the skin
Cocktail chipolata sausage	Sausage roll
Diet drinks, sparkling water, flavoured waters, unsweetened fruit juice, tomato juice	Sugary soft drinks
Fresh fruit salad, ice cream, fruity pudding, thin slices of Brie and Camembert with grapes and oatcakes, a couple of after-dinner mints	Rich dessert, cheese and biscuits, rich chocolates

Hummus, guacamole and wholemeal pitta bread	Cream cheese and white bread
Slowly sipped wine interspersed with water	Wine by the bottle
Smoked salmon with mustard (try recipe for Posh Fish Fingers with Tartare Sauce)	Fried fish goujons, fried scampi, etc.
Spritzer using one measure of spirits and a low-calorie mixer	Neat spirits
Sweet-and-sour dips, tomato-based sauces, yoghurt-based dips, low-fat fromage frais	Mayonnaise and creamy dips
Tangy accompaniments: lemon juice, lime juice, vinegar, acidic dressings and sauces (the acid helps to lower GI)	Sugary stuff: sweet drinks, sugar-rich desserts,etc. (sugar can raise GI)
Tiger prawns with fresh lemon (try recipe for Tiger Prawns with Creamy Dipping Sauce)	Battered crispy prawns
Vegetable crudités and yoghurt dips	Breadsticks with sour cream dip
Vinaigrette dressing, fat-free dressings	Oily dressings
White wine spritzer, 1 medium glass (65 ml wine; 60 ml sparkling water)	Red wine, 1 medium glass (125 ml/4 fl oz)
Your low-GiP carbs: pasta, rice, couscous, grainy breads, potato salad (cold cooked potatoes have a lower GI than hot!), sourdough bread	High-GiP carbs: standard white breads, risotto rice, rice cakes, French fries, pastry

SNACK SWAPS

Enjoy this...	*Because you don't need this...*
Dried fruits	Sugary sweets
Fruity smoothie made from low-fat yoghurt and fresh fruit	Thick sugary milkshake with artificial flavourings
Fruity yoghurt or fromage frais, lower-fat chocolate mousse, reduced-fat rice pudding	Rich dessert
Handful of nuts	Packet of crisps
Home-roasted nuts	Fried and roasted nuts, Bombay Mix
Mini crispbreads, baked crisps	Fried crisps, even vegetable ones – unless they are baked
Mini portions of cheese, reduced-fat feta	Chunk of Cheddar
Oatcake with peanut butter or low-fat soft cheese	Sweet biscuits
Skinny latte, reduced-fat hot chocolate or milkshake	Full-fat milky drinks

TOP TIPS FOR TEMPTING TIMES

You want to have fun and let your hair down. And why not? But party time is when you are most likely to be off your guard and overindulge without thinking. Here is a treasure chest of hot tips that will help you to get through the party feeling slick and chic.

PARTY TRICKS

✳ Eat before you go to the party. This might sound mad, but it will prevent you from arriving there ravenous, ready to attack the buffet table. Choose something low-GI before you leave home – anything from a banana to peanut butter on toast.

✳ If going by car, park the car further away. Walking to the party door will not only help you to burn up some energy, it will also get your blood circulating so that you can be even more alert and energised to enjoy the evening ahead.

✳ Talk more, eat less. Enjoy conversations, meet new people. You might be amazed at some of the party conversations you get into. Chatting more means you're likely to focus on having fun, not having calories.

✳ Pace yourself when it comes to alcohol. The more you drink the less likely you are to keep your resolve to eat sensibly. Try to alternate alcohol with water or unsweetened juice, but remember to avoid sugary soft drinks.

✳ Buffet food is often fried, but there are plenty of healthy alternatives. Go for chicken without the skin dipped in sweet and sour sauce, rather than a drumstick dipped in sour cream.

✳ Drink lots of water. What's stopping you filling your wine glass up with sparkling water?

✳ Dance more, sit less. The more energy you use up, the more fat gets burnt and the shapelier you will begin to look.

✳ Walk tall, stand confident. Try our flatter stomach stance to improve your posture and flatten that tummy immediately. Pull in your stomach muscles tightly, stand as tall as you can, with your shoulders back, chest up and head high. Try it out in the mirror. Good posture can give you an air of confidence. Do this soon after you leave home, and frequently at the party. Be aware of how you're standing even when you're in the depths of a gripping conversation. You never know who might be watching!

🌰 *Put cutlery down between mouthfuls*

WHAT'S IN SOME TYPICAL SNACK FOODS?

This is our Ready Reckoner to show you at a glance how your snack foods stack up on the health scales. We give you typical foods, their calorie value and then what it means in terms of sugar and fat. And, just for fun (and a bit of visual impact!), we've translated the amounts of sugar and fat into sugar cubes and teaspoons of oil. This doesn't literally mean that the food has that many teaspoons of oil; it's just a way of depicting the fat content so you can make a comparison.

Food	Serving	Calories	Equivalent sugar content*	Equivalent fat content**
Café latte	1 medium takeaway (300 ml)	180	▢▢ (40 calories)	**2 tsp** (90 calories)
Chocolate bar	Standard-size bar (65 g)	307	▢▢▢▢▢▢▢▢▢ (180 calories)	**2 tsp** (90 calories)
Croissant	1 medium (60 g)	224	negligible	**2 tsp** (90 calories)
Doughnut	1 medium jam (75 g)	252	▢▢▢ (60 calories)	**2 tsp** (90 calories)
Flapjack	1 medium takeaway (60 g)	296	▢▢▢▢ (80 calories)	**3 tsp** (135 calories)
Milkshake	1 medium takeaway (300 ml)	264	▢▢▢▢▢▢▢ (140 calories)	**1 tsp** (45 calories)
Packet of crisps	Standard-size bag (40 g)	212	negligible	**3 tsp** (135 calories)

* 5 g sugar cubes   ** 1 tsp of oil

Peanuts	I small bag roasted and salted (50 g)	301	none	**5 tsp** (225 calories)

* 5 g sugar cubes   ** I tsp of oil

Have you thought about replacing half your snacks with an alternative containing less sugar and less saturated fat, and more nutritious calories? Here are some ideas…

Food	Serving	Calories	Equivalent sugar content*	Equivalent fat content**
Almonds	12 almonds	159	none	**2 tsp** (90 calories) (healthy fats)
Apple	I medium (100 g/4 oz)	47	▢▢ (40 calories)	negligible
Cereal bar	I medium bar (30 g)	110	▢▢ (40 calories)	**I tsp** (45 calories)
Hummus salad sandwich	Granary bread open sandwich (95 g)	143	negligible	**I tsp** (45 calories)
Minestrone soup	I medium bowl (225 g/8 oz)	68	negligible	**½ tsp** (23 calories)
Oat biscuits	2 medium biscuits (26 g)	122	▢ (20 calories)	**I tsp** (45 calories)
Pineapple	I medium portion (50 g/2 oz)	21	▢ (20 calories)	negligible
Satsuma	I medium (75 g/3 oz)	25	▢ (20 calories)	negligible

* 5 g sugar cubes   ** I tsp of oil

❧ 'Over the past few months, I have lost one stone [6 kg]. In addition, I am now paying more attention to portion control and, most days, I manage the five fruit and veg principle. On the days when I don't, or lapse for whatever reason, I don't beat myself up. I just treat tomorrow as a fresh and positive new beginning. Without the shift in my identity first, I would not have found the sheer determination and commitment to succeed. This is without a doubt, the real key to success.'

HAVE A CRACKING CHRISTMAS

By applying a few simple tips you'll actually get more enjoyment from your festive fayre and come out the other side feeling great.

* Enjoy your turkey, ham and bacon, but avoid the fatty bits. They are great low-fat meats, but remove the skin, visible fat and rind.
* Devour roasted vegetables but spray rather than douse them in oil and cook apart from your meats.
* For snacks before the big meals offer lots of yummy Christmas fruits and lower-fat cheeses like Brie and Camembert along with some tasty breads.
* Serve plenty of delicious brightly coloured vegetables, fruits and salads with your Christmas dinner.
* Fill up on lots of zesty fruits – fresh fruit on a pavlova, citrus fruit kebabs, fruit punch drinks and fruit cocktails.
* Remind yourself of how uncomfortable it feels to be bloated after you've stuffed yourself full of food. It's far

> better to pace yourself and to enjoy eating a fantastic meal
> than to overindulge and feel like you can't get off the sofa.
>
> ✳ If you find you've over-done the alcohol, drink plenty of chilled
> water to re-hydrate yourself, especially if it's a warm day.
>
> ✳ Try going for a post-lunch family walk to blow out the
> cobwebs.
>
> ✳ Don't feel guilty about having treats at Christmas, it's only
> one day and you can always plan a nice light healthy meal
> for Boxing Day to make up for it, with lots of delicious salads
> and leftover lean meats.

The traditional Christmas day meal is packed with further
hidden benefits. Roast turkey without skin is high in protein and
low in fat with only 150 calories in an average portion; potatoes
provide lots of vitamin C as well as fibre. Following the main
course, custard is a warming, high-calcium and low-fat alternative to brandy butter. Nuts are a good source of unsaturated fat
and the antioxidant vitamin E, while dates provide fibre, potassium and iron. As a treat, smoked salmon is an excellent source
of omega-3 fats – good for heart health. And remember, 1 to 2
units of your favourite tipple a day (such as one or two glasses
of wine) may also protect against heart disease.

12 GREAT REASONS TO ENJOY CHRISTMAS FAYRE

✳ Smoked salmon. This tasty treat provides only 80 calories
per portion, and is a good source of protein and the health-
promoting omega-3 fats. Ideal as a starter.

✳ Roast turkey. Rich in protein and low in fat, especially if you
discard the skin and choose light-coloured meat – only 150
calories in an average portion (a couple of slices).

✳ Potatoes. A delicious source of vitamin C and other nutrients. If roasting, use vegetable oil rather than lard to cut saturated fat.

✳ Brussels sprouts. An average serving (9 sprouts) provides half of our daily needs for folic acid and all of our vitamin C.

✳ Carrots. Rich in beta-carotene, which is converted to vitamin A in the body, and carotenoids, which act as potential disease-beating antioxidants.

✳ Peas. Popular with the kids and a good source of iron, zinc, vitamin E, fibre, folic acid and most other B vitamins.

✳ Bucks Fizz. In moderation (1–2 glasses per day), any type of alcoholic drink may help protect against heart disease. And the orange juice adds vital vitamin C.

✳ Christmas pudding. The dried fruit gives plenty of potassium, and it's a reasonable provider of iron and fibre.

✳ Custard. A comforting and low-fat alternative to brandy butter, and a good source of calcium too.

✳ Walnuts. A great source of unsaturated oils and the antioxidant vitamin E. Recent studies suggest the health benefits of being a regular nut eater.

✳ Satsumas. Each of these handy stocking fillers provides half your daily need for vitamin C.

✳ Chestnuts. The only low-fat nut in existence and great for roasting by the fireside.

HEALTHY HOLIDAY EATING

ON THE PLANE...

✳ Remember that some airlines offer low-fat meals but you may need to pre-order this when you book your ticket.

✳ You could take a low-GI sandwich with you, especially since many low-budget flights don't offer complimentary food. Try peanut butter and banana – it will help you to get to your destination feeling ready to enjoy the sights rather than head for the local *boulangerie*!

✳ Skip the complimentary snacks if you order a drink on the plane as these tend to be high in calories.

✳ Even if drinks on the flight are free, don't use this as an excuse to party on free booze.

✳ Avoid taking extra snacks on the flight with you – you are unlikely to go hungry and if you do, well, when was the last time you truly felt hunger pangs?

AT THE RESORT...

✳ Whether self-catering or an all-inclusive holiday this is a good time to try new foods and different ways of cooking. You may even discover new ingredients that you can include in your healthy routine when you get back home. Buy some local dried herbs and spices to take back with you so you can experiment with absent friends!

✳ If you are on an all-inclusive holiday, you don't have to eat as much food as you can each mealtime, just because it's paid for. What will you gain except weight?

✳ If you have a long, leisurely lunch then try to have a lighter evening meal. Similarly, if you think you will be having a substantial evening meal then opt for a light lunch. However, try not to skip any meals, otherwise you're likely to eat more at the earliest opportunity.

✳ Whenever you eat, try to follow the same eating principles you would use at home – remember our VV P C plate model (see page 63), avoid fried food or anything cooked in oil, eat plenty of fresh fruit and vegetables, include low-GI starchy foods such as seeded bread, whole grains and pasta, and avoid fatty and sugary foods and those in rich creamy sauces.

* Many holiday resorts specialise in local fish dishes so take advantage of this and indulge in plenty of fish (grilled, not fried) – it's relatively low in calories and fat. Try experimenting with more unusual seafood such as crabs, oysters, langoustines, fresh sardines, swordfish, etc. They're often much cheaper than back home and you get a chance to try something new.

* Don't be tempted to keep refilling your glass with fruit juice as each glass contains approximately 50 calories. Drink bottled water instead.

* Try to keep some healthy snacks in your room in case you get hungry between meals. Fresh fruit, dried fruit, raw veggies are all good to keep handy.

* If you are served buffet-style food at your hotel, try not to go back for seconds unless these are salad, vegetables and fruit.

* Enjoy continuing with some kind of exercise regime. Exploring new places on foot is a great and inexpensive way to get around, all the while burning the cals!

AT THE RESTAURANT AND BAR...

* Ask for low-calorie/lower-fat varieties of foods like spreads, milk, yoghurt and cheese.

* Nibble on olives instead of other bar snacks as they have less than 5 calories each.

* When ordering salads, ask the waiter for the dressing on the side, or go for a yoghurt- or lime-juice-based one rather than a dressing drenched in olive oil (1 teaspoon of olive oil sets you back nearly 50 calories!).

* Try not to be tempted to drink more alcohol than you would at home. In restaurants ask for a jug of iced water and drink a glass of this between each alcoholic drink.

✳ You can try every item on the menu but you don't have to do it all at once. Try varying your combinations, such as a starter and main course on some days, main course and dessert on others but not all three courses at once.

✳ Choose fresh fruit or fruit salad for dessert if possible.

🐾 Eat out, but avoid creamy sauces and fried dishes

While enjoying your well-deserved break, keep your thinking upbeat and motivated by reminding yourself of just how great you feel, having shed some extra weight and/or inches. This will help you to keep up the good work in terms of being mindful about what you eat and how much you drink.

TAKE IT AWAY? NO, ENJOY IT!

If you're watching what you eat there's no reason why you can't still have takeaway food. Here are some tips to help you choose the healthiest options.

✳ Italian food is not just about pizza and pasta. Many restaurant menus also feature grilled meats, chicken and seafood dishes, which can be ordered with plenty of fresh vegetables.

✳ Pasta has a low glycaemic index, which means it's a great food. It's the sauces that are served with it that can be laden with fat and calories. Order pasta with a fresh tomato sauce – these tend to be lower in fat than cream based ones – and say no to Parmesan cheese! Fill half your plate with the pasta and the other half with fresh local salads.

✳ Go for thin-based pizzas with masses of vegetable toppings and steer clear of extra cheese and processed pepperoni.

* Indian cuisine can be fairly healthy, just be aware of the high-fat fried foods and heavy, butter-based sauces.

* Opt for chicken, prawn or vegetable dishes rather than lamb or beef, which tend to be higher in fat. You might see an orange layer of oil on the top – scoop your serving from underneath.

* Go for tandoori chicken or chicken tikka as they're usually roasted in a tandoor oven, which means they cook quickly without any added fat.

* When it comes to rice, stick to boiled rice and mint raita as a cooling accompaniment.

* If you fancy a Chinese choose healthy starters like satay dishes with chilli dipping sauce, or soups. Avoid anything deep fried, like seaweed and spring rolls.

* When going Thai, stir-fried dishes are a great option as this method of cooking uses very little oil, and look out for dishes with added vegetables.

* Also pick anything on the menu that's steamed, such as whole fish with ginger, steamed vegetables and rice.

FOOD ON THE GO

Fast-food restaurants and cafés spell trouble if you want to eat healthily, but it doesn't mean they're out of bounds. Here are some tips for finding healthy fast food.

* When only a burger will do, look for wholemeal buns – they do exist, and remember that words like jumbo, giant, deluxe and super-sized mean larger portions, larger hips! Order a regular burger and masses of salad – but avoid the dressing unless it's fat-free.

✳ Flavour your burger with sweet-and-sour or tomato sauce and say no to cheese.

✳ Veggie doesn't necessarily mean virtuous. The burgers are generally still cooked in fat, are often high in salt, and served with a creamy sauce.

✳ Try to avoid the temptation of chips. Thin-cut chips like French fries absorb more fat than thick ones, as there's a greater surface area for the oil to seep in to.

✳ If you must have them, remember a regular portion instead of a large could save you half the calories.

✳ Wherever you buy them from, sandwiches are a quick and easy fast-food option. Avoid creamy fillings.

✳ Kebabs can also be healthy and filling as long as the meat is lean. Avoid doner kebabs though – have you seen the fat drip down and congeal at the bottom? Shish kebab is better because the chunks of meat are leaner to start with and are char-grilled, which allows the fat to drain off. Have them in pitta bread stuffed with salad.

✳ For a veggie option, rather than deep-fried falafel, go for a char-grilled vegetable kebab, flavoured with chilli sauce. Pile this into a pitta bread with salad and indulge, safe in the knowledge that you've gone for the healthier option.

✳ If you do find yourself in the chip shop here's my advice. Order a small portion of chips and be careful what you eat them with. Make them into a chip butty with some granary bread, ketchup and salad. Or share them!

✳ If you have fish, get rid of the batter and just eat the fish inside. Or how about having fewer chips and filling up with a pickled egg or pickled onions instead?

AND FINALLY...

* Baked potatoes are a filling, healthy, low-calorie food — it's what you put in them that makes them fattening.

* Ask for no butter and go for healthy fillings like baked beans, chilli con carne with kidney beans, tuna and sweetcorn without the mayo, or cottage cheese and salad.

* In a sandwich bar go for bread that has seed or grains in it and ask for no butter.

* Choose lower-fat fillings such as lean meat, chicken or fish with piles of crunchy salad.

* Say no to mayo and other high-fat accompaniments. Instead go for freshly ground black pepper, mustard, pickles, chutney, salsa or lemon juice to add extra flavour.

CHAPTER NINE:
GOOD WORK – KEEP IT UP!

Every day brings you new choices. All aspects of your life are being shaped by the decisions you make today. The most effective way to get what you desire in the future is to make conscious choices in line with your outcome, in the present.

Think of life as a building process and the accumulative effect that builds up. You will already be delighted with your efforts over the past few days or weeks. The healthy lifestyle that you are now living is becoming second nature. Now build on this. As you let go of old unwanted habits, you make room for new uplifting possibilities.

KEEPING YOUR HOT BODY FOREVER

So you've been on lots of diets, so you've lost lots of weight. But hey, no doubt that weight has just crept back on again. This classic yo-yo dieting does your health no good and doesn't do much for your self-confidence either. You've worked hard to get that hotter body, now's your chance to hang on to it.

❧ *Give compliments and mean it!*

BELIEVE IN YOUR OWN POWER

Imagine for a moment that you have two brains, the thinker and the prover. As you think your thoughts, your prover brain will go all-out to deliver what it is that you are expecting, be it negative or positive. Either way, it will prove you right, this is otherwise known as the self-fulfilling prophecy! For example, if someone believes they are unlikely to achieve a goal, their actions will be consistent with this belief. The prover brain likes to prove it's always right. Therefore your goal for the future to remain healthy, slim, trim, confident and full of energy will be driven by the way you think of yourself and your belief in knowing that you will succeed. This is an example of a positive self-fulfilling prophecy.

Use the following motivational booster as frequently as you choose, to keep on track.

✴ Allow yourself some quiet unrushed time before you begin. Think of a time in the future. It may only be a couple of months or a year or so down the road. Step into this future space as if it were today.

✴ Imagine yourself exactly as you would most like to be. You're being who you really are and doing all the things that you were born to do. You'll know what these are as they'll feel effortless. See yourself surrounded by the people you most wish to be with. In this future place, you'll have taken the most appropriate action in every aspect of your life to make it as magical as it is. How is your life different, richer and more inspiring?

✴ Imagine you can replay the movie backwards and notice what specific actions you took to achieve what you have succeeded in achieving. Remember to notice what motivated you towards success. You may find it easier to run the movie in small frames and only move on when you are crystal clear.

In effect you are giving your prover brain instructions and pictures to guide you to that time in the future.

Above all else, love yourself for who you really are and others will too!

❧ Do a good deed

STEP ONE

Keep up the physical activity. This is now your new, active lifestyle. If you can, throw in another 10-minute chunk of activity whenever you can, so you're now exceeding our original 140 minutes a week activity schedule. The more calories you burn up in activity, the more likely you are to keep your Hot Body. Continue to use our Daily Activity Chart (see page 133) so that you give yourself a tick as a handy motivator.

STEP TWO

You've got used to the Hot Body GiP way of eating, you like it, and it keeps you full and keeps you nourished. So why stop? All you need to do now is to allow yourself slightly larger portions of the healthy lower GI choices until you find you're not losing weight, but just maintaining it. If you are continuing to lose weight, allow yourself a little more. If you start gaining, then just cut back. Remember the golden rules of variety and choosing wisely so that you continue to enjoy health benefits. If you prefer a system where you can count your GiPs and gradually increase the number of GiPs daily, then check out our previous books. You can get a full listing of the GiP value of Gi-tested foods from our original *The Gi Plan* and *The 10-Day Gi Diet.*

> 🍋 *Take up a new interest or hobby*

STEP THREE

As if you needed to be reminded, do refer back to this book from time to time to energise your senses and keep your motivation on track. Continue to try out the mental exercises and visualisations as they will help to keep you focused on a long-term healthier vision of you.

If your goal is to be 5 kg (10 lb) lighter, think, 'Shed ½ kg (1 lb) ten times!' (or adjust to your specific goal). Every food choice you make and the exercise you do on a daily basis, builds up the accumulative effect. So, over the next few weeks, always keep the end result in mind – a mental picture of the ideal new you. Your imagination is by far your greatest tool.

> 🍋 *Accept compliments with just a thank you*

THE LUCKY TOUCH

Who needs a lucky talisman? To stay feeling great about yourself, surround yourself with good company and believe that everything you set your mind to will work out well. The new healthy you is a prime example. Notice then, how good fortune starts to follow you around! Here are some poignant reminders.

GET YOUR MIND ON YOUR SIDE

Whatever you focus on will attract your attention more. If you've been thinking about changing your car, isn't it curious how many of your chosen model, make and colour you keep seeing! Where did they all suddenly come from? Well, of course, they've always been there but up until this time, your attention has been elsewhere. Similarly, when you think about what it is you really want, you increase the likelihood of achieving it as you notice and act more on the opportunities that come your way. Think good fortune, think success, think yourself lucky – and you will be!

> 🐾 'One of my greatest pleasures is walking my dog over the South Downs, headed towards the sea, which we do when I'm working from home. The joy of watching him run and play is childlike and a magical reminder that the simple things in life are free! It's also a powerful reconnection for me with that wonderful sense of freedom both mentally and physically. I return from these brisk walks a lighter soul, having shed any cares and woes along the way and with raised levels of fitness, energy and an overall sense of wellness.'

YOU COUNT, CELEBRATE

Celebrating your successes along the way as you achieve even the smallest of steps towards a goal is an important factor. It will help you in remaining motivated and upbeat about continuing the process. Your achievements come from your ability to 'go for it', so be proud of what you have achieved. Perhaps you can keep a chart or journal? This way, not only can you boost your motivation levels when you need to, but looking back will also remind you that your attitude of 'I can do anything I choose', is there for the taking when you set your mind to it. For example, you're looking and feeling great in your special number because you've stuck to your healthy food plan and regular healthy exercise. Over time, your list will grow, as will your awareness, as you add to life's positives.

LOOK THE PART

Remain open to the good things in life and you're more likely to experience them. Lucky people look the part. They carry themselves in a certain way. Notice their posture and gestures. They're sure to include good eye contact and a lovely smile. Your mind and body are closely linked and making a change in one area will automatically have an influence on the other. So, for example, the way you carry yourself and move about will determine whether your brain releases anxious, stressful chemicals, or happy ones. You choose! Stand tall and be counted. Exude confidence and others will respond accordingly, in a positive way. People respond to you in whichever way you've trained them to do so, be it consciously or unconsciously.

> ❧ *If life looks bleak, get ready to celebrate, you may nearly be home!*

ATTACH YOURSELF TO A LUCKY STAR

Whatever area it is that you wish to strengthen, think of someone who already has these qualities – your personal lucky star – and choose them as your role model. Pay attention to how they do it and then adapt what you learn to suit you, with the relevant tweaks, so you continue to be yourself.

Take an open and honest look at the company you keep. Who you mix with has a big influence on you. Right now, are you mixing with active people, friends who care about their health, diet and fitness? Choose your friends wisely. Present yourself to the world as you would most like to be perceived. Look, sound and feel the part and your actions will become consistent with the way in which you think about yourself.

AND FINALLY...

✳ Think balance. It's not just about GI. The GiP System helps you to incorporate much more than just GI.

✳ Expect your progress to vary. Research suggests that after four to five weeks of steady weight loss, you might even increase in weight by about a pound, or at least plateau. However, this is just your metabolism adjusting. Look at the big picture. If your overall weight is going down, that's success.

✳ Try these craving curbers. Raw courgette wedges are far more substantial and interesting than a celery stick. Cook a whole corn on the cob in the microwave with a couple of tablespoons of water, five sprays of oil and a drizzle of lemon juice. Have the corn GiP-free by using baby corn on the cob from a can. Cook button mushrooms in the microwave with a touch of garlic and dried herbs. Make a refreshing drink with crushed ice, sugar-free cordial and sparkling water. Or make the drink with tap water, freeze it and have as ice cubes or ice lollies.

✳ Enjoy your full allowance of low-GI carbs such as seeded bread, wholegrain cereals, al dente pasta and new potatoes in their skins. Watch the amount of fat you use: choose lower-fat spreads, dairy products, sauces and dressings.

CHAPTER TEN: QUESTIONS AND ANSWERS

I've tried many diet books, how do I really know this is not just another fad (here today gone tomorrow) diet on the market?

When you buy a car, do you get a feel for the honesty of the dealer? Well, when you buy a diet book, gauge the credentials of the authors. Trust in only those who are professionals and who have sound experience and backing. Registered Dietitians are governed by a strict code of conduct, so if an author (as for this book) is a registered dietitian, that's a stamp of quality. Look for the letters RD after the name.

How long before I can expect to see/feel/hear results?

The effects will be almost immediate as long as you've stuck to your Hot Body Plan. Each day counts as part of the accumulative effect and by the end of the week, we would expect you to have lost up to 1 kg (2 lb), which is the safe and sustainable amount that we encourage.

Can I still go out to eat? If so, what can I order at an Indian/Chinese/Italian/French restaurant?

The beauty of GiP is that you can continue to enjoy eating out, one of the little pleasures of life (see pages 192–4).

What if friends ask me to dinner? Do I warn them in advance what I can/can't eat? If I stop the diet when I'm, for example, on holiday, will all my good work be undone?

Nothing is out of bounds, just be mindful of your daily allowance of food. For the same reason, being on holiday means that you can continue to eat well by choosing your foods in line with the GiP System (see pages 189–92).

Do I have to buy lots of expensive foodstuffs?

No. The fab thing about how this diet works is that you can buy what is within your budget. Our advice is to buy the best food you can that suits your pocket.

Do I have to keep count or track of saturated fat and calories?

No – we keep track of the GiPs and take care of the calories. It's easy because we've done all the complicated maths for you. All you do is keep to the V V P C rule. Simple as 1–2–3!

Can kids and old people safely follow this diet?

Yes, with the guidance of a Registered Dietitian so that the portion sizes are right for the age group.

How safe is this diet in terms of cholesterol?

The foods recommended in the GiP System are designed to be lower in fat, especially saturated fat that has a strong influence on your blood cholesterol. It is always best to seek the advice of your GP if you have any medical conditions before starting any diet.

Will I feel tired when I first start the diet?

You might find that you've never felt better! This isn't a fad diet, which restricts your calories to very low levels. Use the guidelines to achieve balance and variety, keep to the portion sizes and see how you go. If you are losing weight too quickly, have a little more of the same healthy foods. Obviously, if you do feel tired or unwell, check with your GP.

How does the Hot Body Plan differ from other diets?

Each diet has it's own guidelines and principles. A diet plan, which incorporates a range of healthy foods from all the main food groups (carbs, proteins, fruit and veg, and dairy foods) plus an exercise recommendation, is a good sign. The Hot Body Plan is based on good principles – and qualified nutritionists and dietitians use GI routinely as a guide to healthy eating.

What sort of real changes will I have to make in my life for this to work?

The real change is making up your mind to make the change and following through on it by taking appropriate action. We have built in highly motivational, tried-and-tested tools, coupled with some 'mental gymnastics' to make it all effortless for you.

Will this diet be detrimental to my system over the long term?

The opposite is true. It will enhance your health and wellbeing through eating in a balanced and healthy way. Just make sure you vary the foods you choose and keep to the guidelines.

If this is so good why has no one else come up with the idea before?

GI has been around for a long time. It just took us to put in the enormous time and effort to prove that, once put into a user-friendly, practical system, it can be used successfully by both men and women.

Will this be an expensive diet to maintain?

No. Its flexibility allows for you to use whatever you usually put aside for your weekly food shop.

How do I maintain my weight once I have lost the pounds?

Good question! This is a lifestyle change, for the better. You simply increase your portion sizes and gauge your weight regularly.

How easy is the diet to do?

It's as easy as pie! We've done all the hard work for you. Simply read what the diet's about and follow our menu-planning advice. If you think it'll be easy, it will and if you don't, it won't!

Will I need to take supplements/nutrients alongside the diet?

The diet is designed to be able to facilitate a range of foods, which will help you achieve all-round good nutrition. However, you might want to take a supplement as a safety net, in case you're not very good at varying what you eat. Only choose a supplement that offers no more than 100 per cent of the RDA of vitamins and minerals.

Can you guarantee that I will lose weight on this diet?

We can't, but *you* can – by following the advice on food choices and physical activity.

What sort of research have you done to ensure it is different from the rest of the diets out there?

The research on GI is extensive, which is why we also include the science behind it from time to time. And that offers you only a fraction of the studies that are out there.

How long will it take me to get down to my ideal weight?
We would recommend that you aim for no more than ½–1 kg (1–2 lb) in a week.

Will I lose weight straight away?
We would expect you to lose at least 1 kg (2 lb) in weight at the end of your first week, providing you have followed our recommendations.

I have been overweight for the last 20 years and have been on many boom-bust diets. How do I know this one is different and won't affect my health?
Many diet books do not offer the uniqueness of our powerful, motivational boosters. Knowledge is not enough unless it is supported by a positive approach and mental attitude, which make the changes in your lifestyle sustainable. Couple this with a diet plan that is compiled by expert dietitians and you're well on your way to a healthier, new you. If you are at all concerned about starting the diet, it is always best to seek the advice of your GP.

How do I prevent myself eating when I'm not really hungry?
The good news about GiP is that you don't feel hungry! And if you do, there are plenty of GiP-free goodies to keep you going. Remember too that distraction works effectively. Take your mind off food by doing something else that you enjoy that is healthy, such as exercise, reading or making a phone call. There are many great tips on this throughout the book.

I am a comfort eater. What can I do to control this?
If it's comfort that you are in need of, find another way of getting this pleasure in a more functional way. Try a bubble bath or meditation.

I eat when I'm bored. What tips can you offer?

It is common to eat when you have a need that is unmet and boredom is one of them. Find other ways to relieve the boredom. There are many suggestions in this book. And if you want to eat, just choose a GiP-free food.

I'm overwhelmed by the changes that I'd need to make to my whole lifestyle to make this work. Is there a quick and easy way?

This diet is designed, along with our tips on exercise, to fit in effortlessly with your lifestyle. By making bite-size-chunk changes daily, you'll accomplish your goal easily.

Sometimes I feel that my body is 'stuck' and sluggish. What practical tips are there?

Physical activity works wonders for the mind and the body, which are linked. It's fab for beating the blues, too. This book contains plenty of tips on this.

I'm not sure that I can handle the expectations that I have about myself when I'm slim. What do you suggest?

You won't know until you've tried. Be that person today, ahead of time. See yourself as the new you and become him/her, as if you've *already* achieved your goal. Now think about what these expectations are and how the new, more confident, energetic you would handle these.

How do I get round not offending my hosts, partner, family, etc. by leaving food on the plate, when I'm full?

Do what you can to make sure that you get served smaller portions, or serve yourself.

How do I stay motivated?
There are loads of motivation and booster tips in this book. Some of them are our best-kept secrets, until now!

How can I raise my level of motivation when it's down?
Think about what achieving this outcome will ultimately do for you and how your life will be different. Follow our motivational tips throughout the book.

Most of my mates eat and drink excessively when we're out. How do I resist the temptations?
Be focused on your outcome, not theirs! There's a satisfaction in knowing that you'll be the one waking up minus that distended tum or blinding headache, not to mention having a mouth that tastes like a parrot's cage!

I feel that I'm so overweight, how do I kick start my motivation?
Take each day as it comes and do whatever it takes in even the smallest of ways to achieve small goals along the way. Keep a desirable picture of you somewhere prominent so you can remind yourself of what the new you will look like.

I feel that my weight is linked with other stuff that is going on in my life. How do I go about sorting this out?
Food fills a physical hole not an emotional need. Understanding what the other stuff is, which clutters your life, is the place to start. Take one issue at a time to simplify and de-clutter your life. We include some of the best guidance, ever!

I'm imaging myself and my life to become very different when I'm the 'right' size. How realistic is this?

The trick here is to enjoy your life as it is in the now. Visualising how you want it to be in the future will increase the likelihood, so make it as ideal as you would wish for.

I've a suspicion that deep down something stops me from wanting to reduce my size. Can you help?

There is a pay off in keeping things as they are. If there wasn't, you would have made the change already. Work out what it is that stops you and with our guidance, build it into your outcome, in a healthy way.

When I am infatuated or fall in love, my appetite is automatically suppressed. How do I avoid ballooning later on in the relationship?

Love and infatuation act as natural suppressants. You're full up with pleasurable feelings, so you tend to eat less. Ballooning later suggests that you are then trying to fill emotional needs with food, which doesn't work. Understand what the emotional needs are, talk these through with your partner and move on.

My partner cooks wonderful meals and gets irritable about my new eating regime. Any tips around dealing with this?

Open communication is the thing. Get your partner on your side, supporting you and who knows, when you help them to find what the value might be to them, too, they may even join in.

I don't eat when I'm stressed and so tend to lose weight, which is great. However, remaining in this state isn't a healthy or functional way to do it. How can I make it easy at other times?

Set about de-stressing your life and look for ways to encourage a healthy flow of energy in and around yourself. Find functional ways to motivate yourself. There are plenty of ideas in this book.

How do I stick with the commitment to get to my 'new me'?
Start by getting really clear about all the benefits that being your new self will bring. Write these down and pin them up. Put up a past photo of yourself or one of an inspirational model. Plan and shop for food as much in advance as you can to make the commitment easier. And, build in a daily exercise routine that effortlessly fits in with your day.

Will the GI diet help me lose those inches?
To date at least 16 studies have examined the effects of GI on appetite and all but one have demonstrated an increase in satiety, delayed hunger return and reduced food intake following the consumption of low-GI foods than following that of high-GI foods.

When can I expect to see the results of a regular exercise regime?
You don't expect the perfect body in a single workout but small cumulative steps mount up fast and effectively. The noticeable changes will come, but be mindful that everyone is different so it will take as long as it takes. Make up your mind to succeed and you will! Some things to look for include: an increase in stamina, muscle definition and dropping a dress size. To keep motivated, find a buddy and write down your workout schedule, weekly. Remember that as little as two 10-minute bursts of moderate physical exercise or 20 minutes in one go, enough to leave you slightly breathless, is our recommended daily guideline.

Why can't I lose weight, when I'm doing everything by the book?
It is said that each individual has an optimum, natural weight. If this tends to be on the heavy side, it will mean increasing your physical activity over time and possibly eating less or eating with more awareness, which could result in the same thing. In your fitness

regime, remember to include manageable cardiovascular training and stretching (for added flexibility), too. Psychologically, many people feel they could do with shedding a few extra pounds or inches, so keep it real. If your main goal is to be healthy and happy, ask yourself if you really need to lose any more.

How can I realistically find time for me, when my days are constantly spent juggling the demands of kids, relationships and work?

No one is saying that it's the easiest thing to do, but it probably is one of the most important. By taking care of yourself you are more likely to take better care of others. In addition, you become a role model – the message says, 'I'm important, too.' You train others to respond and treat you in the way that you would wish, so you may as well do it positively as opposed to saying, 'It's alright to use me as the doormat!'

What would be an instant 'fix-it' to enhance my appearance?

Get an instant 'wow!' by standing up straighter, pulling in your tummy muscles. The illusion is of an immediate loss of several pounds, which in turn often acts as a powerful motivational booster to stick to or start a 'new you' goal.

How do I maintain my efforts during the Christmas and New Year party season?

The challenge, especially during this period, affects even the die-hard! The combination of eat more and exercise less, due to demands on your time, can result in gaining a few pounds but doesn't have to be a foregone conclusion. With a tad of extra discipline around your planning, you can come near or still achieve your required workout. There are party season food tips to support you in this book. And, if you do fall off the wagon, enjoy the moment for what it is. As mad as that may sound, it is likely to make you more determined to get back on the straight and narrow! Each day brings new beginnings.

What actually happens in my body when I eat the low-GI way?

'Whole foods', such as whole grains, and foods that are high in 'soluble fibre', such as soya beans, will take longer to be broken down by the body and will thus cause a slower rise in blood glucose. If you imagine how easy it is to digest some puréed pea soup — it's already in small particles (and quite sloppy, though delicious!). It would make sense to suggest that the body does- n't need to mash this up for too long before the soup is digested and ready to go into the bloodstream as glucose. Now imagine how much longer it would take for you to digest whole peas.

The body needs to break down the skin before it even reaches the pulp of the peas, then it needs to break that down into a mush before it is small enough to enter the bloodstream. So, the whole peas will make the blood glucose rise much slower than the puréed soup. This is the case with most foods — hummus compared to a whole-chickpea casserole, mashed potatoes compared to a jacket potato, and wholemeal bread compared to seeded bread.

Why do low-GI foods keep us full for longer?

If you like your facts, you may want to know that when the blood glucose level rises, the body responds by releasing a hormone, insulin, from the pancreas. This process is called insulin response. Insulin transports the glucose from the blood to either muscle or fat stores to be used as energy. This then reduces the blood glucose level. The faster a food raises blood glucose levels, the greater the insulin response. This results in a rapid fall in blood glucose again, and this is associated with hunger. So, the more you eat foods that cause a slow rise in blood glucose, the less hungry you are likely to feel.

Glucose also comes from other foods, but mainly from the starchy and sugary foods you eat. With new scientific evidence, we now know that all carbohydrate foods do not have the same effect on blood glucose. The amount and type of fat, the type of fibre and even the way food is cooked or processed is more important.

CHAPTER ELEVEN: QUICK GUIDE TO THE HOT BODY PLAN

B y now we hope you will have been convinced that getting the Hot Body you want is achievable. Now we want to show that it's as easy as ABC! In this concluding section we give you an alphabetical round-up of the salient points of the Hot Body Plan, both to remind you of what we have talked about and to really drive the message home. Use this section as a memory jogger and a morale booster when your motivation is starting to lag.

IT'S AS EASY AS A B C!

A IS FOR ACTIVITY

A daily dose of physical activity can set you well on the way to the Hot Body you want. Build in at least 20 minutes of exercise each day. Choose an activity that's so much fun it's effortless, and fit it in to your normal lifestyle so that you won't even notice. Variety is the spice of life, so try all kinds of interesting and unusual activities! Recruit your partner, friend, kids or the dog as exercise buddies for motivation and inspiration.

🐾 *Use it or lose it!*

B IS FOR BED

A good night's rest is essential. Your body has a natural cycle of sleep. It knows when to sleep. Make sure your bed is associated with sleep. Don't lie there chatting on the phone, watching TV or doing anything else that keeps the brain alert and active. If you can't get to sleep after 40 minutes or so, get up and do something really boring until you get drowsy.

C IS FOR CONGRATULATIONS!

Congratulate yourself every small step of the way. This is what you'd do to encourage a toddler to walk. Be that toddler today! Rewards come in different packages, but the best are the words of support you say to yourself, just as if you were encouraging someone else. Every week, to support yourself with your new 'you' goal, congratulate yourself as you swap old habits for new. Choose the stairs instead of the escalator – 'Well done!' Give that doughnut a miss – 'Brilliant!' Check the tone, volume and energy in your voice as you offer these positive words of congratulations.

Celebrate every success no matter how small

D IS FOR 'DON'T SAY DIET'

If you say to yourself you must avoid a food, you'll crave it even more! Just saying 'diet' conjures up other 'D' words like deprivation and despair! Challenge your thinking about food. Know which foods are low GiP/low calorie and choose more of them. You can still have high-GiP/high-calorie choices – just less often. There's a place for all types of food.

E IS FOR ELEPHANTS!

If you think about elephants, they'll pop up everywhere! What has this got to do with getting a Hot Body? Everything! If you can dream it, you can make it happen! Thomas Edison dreamed he could light up the world and 10,000 tries later, he succeeded. Imagine how you'd love the 'Hot' you to look. Now, see yourself doing all the things you'd most love to try and sharing them with the people that matter most. Feel your confidence grow. Enjoy the surge of energy. Soak up that on-top-of-the-world feeling.

& *Dare to dream!*

F IS FOR FOOD ALTERNATIVES

Food can fill a physical void but not an emotional one. The comfort you seek needs to be provided in a better way than through comfort eating. Regain control and experiment with new and healthier ways. For example, if you find that meditation is as comforting as unhealthy snacking, choose meditation! Or, if you find a chat with a mate is uplifting and you don't need the ice cream any more, then pick up the phone!

G IS FOR GI – AND GLUCOSE

The speed at which carbohydrate foods are digested plays an important part in your overall health. Different carbs raise blood glucose at different rates. Low-GI foods cause slow, gradual rises and help you manage your weight. High-GI carbs cause quick, sharp rises so don't eat these on their own. That's the principle of GI. But GI alone is not enough. Hence the Hot Body Plan's GiP System – a balanced plan for healthy eating!

H IS FOR HOT! HOT! HOT!

Here are some Hot! Hot! Hot! tips to burn off those calories. Build exercise into your daily schedule. When you can't get to a pool, tone up with a brisk walk up and down the stairs. Park your car 10 minutes from your destination and walk briskly the rest of the way. Take the stairs and not the lift. While the kettle's boiling, try some stretching exercises, jogging on the spot or even sit-ups. Or just put on some music and dance!

I IS FOR INFLUENCE

Mind and body are linked. A change in one area influences the other. Think happy thoughts and you'll release happy chemicals. Think stressful thoughts and you'll release stress chemicals. Your thoughts are reflected in your physiology and show in what you say and do. Make your mind work for you.

> ❧ *Mind and body are inextricably linked*

J IS FOR JUICE

Enjoy a glass of unsweetened fruit juice daily with a meal so the other bits of your meal are digested with the juice, helping you achieve nice slow, steady blood sugar rises.

K IS FOR KEEPING ON AN EVEN KEEL

If you are on the hamster wheel of life, spinning round and round, not knowing where you'll end up, it's time to press the emergency stop button. Get back on an even keel by nourishing yourself mentally, emotionally and physically. Keep centered and balanced and you'll make healthy choices. Be grateful for all you have – and for all you don't have, too!

L IS FOR LAUGHTER

You can't get enough! Laughter helps combat stress. Children laugh 400 times a day. Adults laugh 20 times a day – if that! Be like a child and brighten up your life and those around you. It's free and it's infectious!

Surround yourself with playful personalities

M IS FOR MOTIVATION

People who think about what they really want and not what they don't want, are more likely to achieve their goal The brain is programmed to give you more of what you focus on and these thoughts expand. Be the bodyguard of your own thinking. Think often about your goal and all the likely benefits, and this will strengthen your motivation.

Believe that you can only succeed

N IS FOR NICE – NOT NAUGHTY

Before you give in to temptation, ask yourself if that choice will take you nearer to the new 'you'. If not, choose again! Food has emotional, psychological and social aspects, so examine your attitude and strike the right balance. If your blood glucose is steady throughout the day, you're more likely to feel on top of things.

O IS FOR ORANGE

Bright coloured foods such as oranges, yellows and reds, have powerful antioxidants to revitalise your skin, hair and immune system. You get these super nutrients from carrots, yellow peppers, sweet potatoes, papaya and many more – eat a rainbow!

P IS FOR PARTY ANIMAL

Your body is a temple, but sometimes it's a nightclub! A little of what you fancy does you good and so does knowing when to

222 * THE HOT BODY PLAN

stop. If you go astray in your healthy food choices or indulge in a glass too many, let it go and enjoy the naughtiness of the lapse. Tomorrow is another day. Make a fresh start.

ࣦ *Today's choices are your future*

Q IS FOR QUALITY AND QUANTITY

It's not about low carb, but slow carb. Choose quality carbs like pasta that are digested slowly. But eat the right quantity, too – enough, but not too much or you'll tip the scales in the wrong direction!

R IS FOR ROUGH

Think about whether a food is rough or smooth. This is a great instant GI assessment for many foods. An apple is rough. Apple juice is smooth. Choose the apple. Potatoes in skins are rough. Mash is smooth. Choose the skins. Granary bread is rough. Wholemeal is smooth. You choose.

S IS FOR SAD

From September to April winter blues – SAD or Seasonal Affective Disorder – affects many people, women in particular. This is caused by a biochemical imbalance due to lack of sunlight. You want to hibernate, can't sleep or sleep all the time, crave sweet things and lose self-esteem. Fight it by getting out in the day, whether or not it's sunny. Keep physically active to boost your feel-good factor and increase self-esteem.

ࣦ *Have a massage*

T IS FOR TRIMMINGS

It's the trimmings on the side of a meal that can clock up the calories and pop the buttons. Creamy sauces, oily dressings, a rasher of bacon around the chicken breast, the fresh cream served with the fruit salad, the list goes on. Christmas trimmings alone probably add 1000 calories. Trim off those trimmings and get trim.

U IS FOR UNISEX AND UNIFORM

The GiP System is for men and women. We recommend you lose a uniform ½–1 kg (1–2 lb) a week, and no more. We want you to *keep* your Hot Body, not *borrow* it. If you are losing more than this amount each week (and this applies especially to men), have slightly larger portions and see what happens. You're the best gauge of your success.

V IS FOR V V P C

Here's a practical visualisation tip to keep you on track with your healthy eating. Imagine you have a couple of chopsticks and you placed them across each other on top of your plate so that the plate is divided into quarters. Fill two quarters with **V**eggies (or salad), one quarter with **P**rotein (meat, fish or pulses) and one quarter with **C**arbs (pasta, rice, potatoes). This way you'll have healthier portions, lower GI and get a range of vitamins and minerals.

W IS FOR WORRY AND WASTE

Your worries will probably never happen and are a waste of energy that could be put to better use. Most worries are about the future, not the present. Live in the moment and don't worry about what might not happen. If your worries are about the past, they're history! Learn and move on. Every problem has a solution. Change your 'don't wants' to 'wants' and take a positive step towards the next day.

🐸 *Live in the now!*

X IS FOR X RATED

It's free and you'll burn up calories! 30 minutes of sexy-cise will lose you around 200 calories. Sex lifts your mood, boosts circulation, reduces tension and tones stomach and thighs. And, if all that isn't enough, you'll live longer, too!

Y IS FOR YES!

Yes, I can do it! You're in control of your life and that includes the choices you make. Adopting a 'yes, I can' attitude is positive and fun. You're far more likely to succeed if you believe you can. 'Yes, I can eat slowly and savour my food', 'Yes, I can choose fruity snacks, not processed junk' and 'Yes, I can get the Hot Body I want!'

Z IS FOR ZEST

Develop a zest for life and live life to the full. Let children be your teachers. They laugh a lot, play a lot and live in the moment. Life is not a dress rehearsal. Live each day as if it were your last performance. Throw caution to the wind. Run barefoot in the park. Roll your trousers up and splash in the waves. Be grateful for all life offers – and be who you were born to be.

FINAL NOTE: HAPPY DAYS!

On a mid-summer's day, soak up the rays and pour yourself a refreshing glass of something cool. As you anticipate that first sip, notice how you feel. Do you describe this feeling as pleasure or happiness? The two are easily confused and although one can produce the other, pleasure is experienced through the enjoyment of the five senses. Pleasure is a great feeling that might come with savouring delicious food, a glass of wine, watching a film, or feeling the sand between your toes on a sandy beach, the wind blowing in your hair. Happiness is independent of objects and events. It is in your soul.

When you are happy, you are less likely to let minor annoyances upset you. When you are unhappy, they're more likely to get to you. You may well find yourself diving into the biscuit barrel or eating sweets to compensate, and get a quick pleasure fix. Sadly, though, the unhappiness remains.

To see the bright fish,
the water must clear.
To see the sun,
the clouds must pass.
Even when hidden,
sun and fish are there.

There is happiness in your soul.
   To reach it you must be still and quiet...

Some people are afraid to experience the happiness factor, at all. They believe they are better off without it, as it is followed by unhappiness, and perhaps, in the extreme, won't seek it at all. However, you are born with a yearning for happiness and your actions, in one way or another, gravitate towards what you believe will help you achieve it. Everyone wants to feel good.

When something happens that alleviates your anxieties or brings a happy outcome, notice how calm your mind becomes. With this kind of mental relaxation, comes a sense of calm, which manifests happiness. When the burden, the worry or fear goes, or you no longer have to strive, chase or pursue the desire, the tension washes away and happiness appears in the form of a feeling that comes from inside. Happiness can be hidden by your clouds of worries and desires, and the endless inner chatter of the mind.

SIGN UP HERE

* Detach yourself from every trivial feeling so that you are not blown in every which direction.
* Remain relaxed and calm.
* Happiness is independent of external events. It is not buried under a rock, so stop searching – you're looking in the wrong place!
* Calm the incessant chatter of your mind and silence the thoughts.
* Bring happy thoughts into all you do and say.

TIPPED TO TOP

Here are some practical tips for you to try out in everyday life. Remember, how you feel is a matter of personal choice. You can choose an attitude of happiness or unhappiness! You do not have control of outside events, people or circumstances but you can choose how you respond. Of course there are many situations that are not conducive to happiness, but you are the bodyguard of your thinking and at any time you can refuse to think about them. Instead, concentrate on the happy moments in time.

* Every problem is a solution waiting to happen.
* Reading inspiring stories daily will uplift you.
* Be grateful for all you have and all you haven't!
* At the end of each day, congratulate yourself for all you've achieved and don't fret about what you didn't get around to.
* Choose funny films, books and people who make you laugh.
* Uplifting music lifts up your spirit.
* Reward yourself in some small way, at the end of each day.
* Expect to enjoy the day, expect to experience happiness and bring it into your thoughts and deeds.
* Be happy for others.
* Extend one small act of kindness, daily. Let someone out in traffic, send a card, buy someone a coffee. Happiness breeds happiness.
* Surround yourself with great company.
* Smile. It will brighten up your day and others, too.
* Practise remaining detached. Accept events outside your immediate control. Whatever the circumstances, they will pass – situations are cyclical. Remain calm and relaxed. Happiness is accessed through peacefulness.

> ✑ 'A daily dose of fresh air provides me with all
> the usual benefits like filling my lungs with oxygen
> and strengthening other organs and muscles, but
> also a lengthy "me moment". Me time means I
> can create, meditate or simply soak up the
> sunshine, when it's out, thereby topping up the
> vitamin D, too! The freshness of this time helps to
> clear away any cobwebs and often provides me
> with answers to things that I had been pondering
> or stuck on!'

A DAY IN THE LIFE OF HAPPINESS

What would it be like if you decided to live one day of your life differently? What if you planned it so that this day would be the most wonderful, enjoyable and satisfying, ever? If you're up for the challenge, here's what you need to plan the night before.

✳ Set your alarm for one hour earlier than usual.
✳ Prepare your mind to accept this by realising all the benefits that this small change will bring.
✳ Regardless of the weather (it's tempting to stay snuggled up under the duvet on a wet, chilly morning), jump out of bed as soon as the alarm goes off or even before it rings and smile!
✳ Put some quality time aside this morning to meditate, even for as little as 10 minutes. Do this using any technique that you choose and if you are not familiar with meditation, simply bring to mind happy experiences from your past. Hang on to the recreation of these happy feelings through-out the day.

DESIGN YOUR DAY – THE CANVAS IS BLANK
Pick 'n' mix from the examples below, or create your own.

* Visualise yourself savouring the day in a calm, peaceful and unhurried manner. Know with confidence that whatever challenges today brings, you'll relish facing them (even look forward to them), knowing that you'll do your personal best. And, remind yourself that today is extra special and wonderful.

* Enjoy a healthy breakfast including foods that you like and that make you feel energised. You've already created the time to savour a leisurely breakfast.

* When you commute today, by car, tube, train or bus, be more respectful of others. Give up your seat to someone who needs it more than you. Let a car out in front of you. Being kind to others will make you feel kinder in yourself and, hopefully, will breed kindness so that others will pass on the good deed.

* As you start your work, carry with you the good intention to smile (a genuine one goes a long way!) and be patient and tolerant. Adopt an attitude of 'can do' and handle each situation in a positive manner. You have an automatic responsibility towards others.

* Increase your awareness around all that you do today. When you eat, focus your wholehearted attention on tasting every morsel. Ditch the juggling. Concentrate on your activities, one at a time, giving each thing, person or conversation your undivided attention by being present in each moment.

* Leave behind the living legacy that you would most wish to be remembered by in all your interactions today. Be it with the butcher, baker or candlestick maker! How would you

most want them to describe you after you leave them? Being polite, considerate and kind is usually free!

✳ It's getting to the close of the day. Time to reward yourself in some small way and have time out, even for a few minutes, for 'me time'. Choose this time alone to spend in any way that helps to nourish your mind, body and/or soul.

✳ Your loved ones and those nearest and dearest are to be treasured. Openly show your appreciation and affection in some small way. A hug, kiss or even a token pressie or card. Enjoy what quality time you have together at the end of a day.

✦ Happiness is a journey not a destination

Today is different and special. Live in the moment. It's a gift. If you felt a positive impact from today's experience, you may choose another wonderful day, tomorrow and the day after.

THE SCIENCE

BENEFITS OF 5 PER CENT WEIGHT LOSS

1. Mertens IL & Van Gaal LF (2000). Overweight, Obesity and Blood Pressure: The Effects of Modest Weight Reduction. *Obesity Research* **8**: 270–8.

This is a review of studies showing that **a modest weight loss of 5 per cent can improve blood pressure levels and reduce the need for medication**. The authors suggest that moderate weight reduction should be considered as a treatment strategy for overweight patients as it is easier to maintain but still has a positive effect on hypertension.

A four-year randomised controlled trial called the Hypertension Control Programme examined the blood pressure levels of patients on medication for raised blood pressure. One group of patients stopped medication and made changes to their diet (reducing calorie and salt intake). Another group, the control group, only stopped taking the medication. Four years later, the dietary group had lost an average of 4.7 per cent (3.8 kg) of their original weight and 39 per cent of the patients had normal blood pressure levels without medication. In contrast, patients in the control group had gained an average of 2 kg and only 5 per cent of the patients had normal blood pressure levels without medication.

Another study, Trials of Hypertension Prevention, showed that **weight loss had a beneficial effect in patients who were at risk of developing hypertension.** Some 308 patients with normal blood pressure readings followed a weight-loss programme. Weight and blood pressure readings were then compared to those of a control group (256 patients) 18 months later. The weight reduction group lost an average of 3.9 kg (4.3 per cent) and their diastolic and systolic blood pressure levels fell by 2.3 mmHg and 2.9 mmHg respectively. The control group had double the amount of patients diagnosed with hypertension compared to the weight reduction group (13.3 per cent vs. 6.5 per cent).

2. Diabetes Prevention Programme Research Group (2002). Reduction in the incidence of type 2 diabetes with lifestyle intervention or metformin. *New England Journal of Medicine* **346**: 393–403

This study found that **losing about 5 per cent of body weight may reduce the risk of developing type 2 diabetes.** Some 3234 subjects were randomly placed in one of three intervention groups. One group were given metformin (a drug used to treat diabetes) and lifestyle advice, the second group were given a placebo and lifestyle advice and the third group followed an intensive weight-loss programme (low-fat, low-calorie diet and 150 minutes of physical activity per week). After three years, the group following the weight-loss programme had lost an average 5.9 per cent (5.6 kg) of their initial weight and had a 58 per cent lower occurrence of diabetes than those who took the placebo. Those on metformin also did better than the placebo group. They lost an average of 2.2 per cent of their initial weight and had a 31 per cent lower incidence of diabetes than the placebo group.

3. Schuler G, Hambrecht R, Schlierf G et al. (1992). Regular Physical Exercise and Low-fat Diet: Effects on Progression of Coronary Artery Disease. *Circulation* **86**: 1–11

In this study it was found that **only a 5 per cent weight loss led to a decrease in cholesterol levels.** Cholesterol leads to plaque build-up in the arteries (atherosclerosis) which is a principal cause of heart disease. This one-year German study, of 113 men, took place in Heidelberg. Half of the sample followed an exercise programme and followed a low-fat, low-cholesterol diet. At the end of 12 months they had lost 5 per cent of their initial weight but their total cholesterol levels had dropped by 10 per cent. In addition, their low-density lipoprotein levels ('bad cholesterol') had fallen by 8 per cent.

4. Pi-Sunyer FX (1993). Short-term Medical Benefits and Adverse Effects of Weight Loss. *Annals of Internal Medicine* **119** (7): 722–6

This review summarises the many effects that weight loss can have. As with the articles above, it also highlights the effect that modest weight loss has on high blood pressure and diabetes. In addition, it points out that **'good cholesterol levels' can be boosted by a 5 per cent loss** of initial weight and conditions like sleep apnoea (air is blocked from getting into the lungs when asleep) can improve. The author also quotes studies that show that small levels of weight loss can reduce hospital stays and complications after surgery. Losing weight can also reduce joint and back pain.

FURTHER INFORMATION

Visit Az and Nina on **www.giplan.com** and **www.thinkwelltobe well.com**

www.giplan.com is a supportive site for anyone wanting to get into low-GI-eating by using the Gi Plan Diet and motivational strategies. If you've already bought the book and need a quick inspirational 'top up', or some new menu ideas, this is worth a visit. For the uninitiated, **www.giplan.com** will simply whet your appetite.

www.thinkwelltobewell.com offers golden nuggets of information and inspires you to check and challenge your thinking, approach and attitudes to food choices and many aspects of life. It offers willpower boosters, slimming tips, and a host of information on diet and diabetes.

Or visit Az on her website: **www.govindjinutrition.com**

If you want to see Az and Nina in action on the web, visit: **https://nutritionandfitness.healthinsurance.tescofinance.com**

BOOKS

The 10-Day Gi Diet by Azmina Govindji and Nina Puddefoot, Vermilion, 2006

The Gi Plan by Azmina Govindji and Nina Puddefoot, Vermilion, 2004

Think Well To Be Well by Azmina Govindji and Nina Puddefoot, Diabetes Research & Wellness Foundation, 2002

EXPERTS

Registered dietitians hold the only legally recognisable graduate qualification in nutrition and dietetics. If you would like to visit a dietitian, contact:

The British Dietetic Association
5th Floor, Charles House
148/9 Great Charles Street
Queensway
Birmingham B3 3HT
Tel: 0121 200 8080

The Diabetes Research & Wellness Foundation (DRWF)
The DRWF is a charity working to relieve the suffering of people with diabetes and related illnesses.

The Diabetes Research and Wellness Foundation
Northney Marina
Hayling Island
Hampshire
PO11 ONH
Tel: 023 9263 7808

OTHER WEBSITES

The British Dietetic Association sites include:
www.bda.uk.com
www.weightwisebda.uk.com

For diabetes-specific sites, visit:
www.diabeteswellnessnet.org.uk
www.diabetes.org.uk

For further information about wholegrains, visit:

www.wholegraingoodness.com

USEFUL WEBSITES FOR MORE INFORMATION ON ALCOHOL

Drink Aware

This website lists common brands of alcoholic drink and will calculate the number of units they contain.

www.drinkaware.co.uk

Other useful sites include:

www.knowyourlimits.gov.uk

www.alcoholconcern.org.uk

www.eatwell.gov.uk/healthydiet/nutritionessentials/drinks/alcohol

Below is an easy guide on the size of measuring spoons and a 200 ml glass.

serving spoon

tablespoon

teaspoon

200 ml glass

INDEX

The Gi Plan
Lose weight forever

The glycaemic index (GI) is one of the hottest topics in dieting today, yet even using that to shed kilos can be difficult. However, with *The Gi Plan* there's no stress and no complicated calculations.

Each food item has been given a value, known as 'GiPs': simply add up the GiPs of your favourite food each day and off you go! And it's flexible – even if you are a bit naughty now and then, you can still lose weight and get healthy.

The 10-Day Gi Diet
Lose up to an inch off your waist

The 10-Day Gi Diet offers a unique system that combines quick but safe weight loss with inspiring tools to help you change your eating habits – for good.

Easier and healthier than other diets,
this eating plan offers you:
- Ultimate flexibility
- Tasty menu choices and recipes
- Motivating ways to change your relationship with food

The 10-Day Gi Diet is a simple, easy-to-follow plan that offers visible results – in just 10 days.

☐ The Gi Plan   9780091900090   £7.99

☐ The 10-Day Gi Diet   9780091906979   £6.99

FREE POSTAGE AND PACKING

Overseas customers allow £2.00 per paperback.

BY PHONE: 01624 677237

BY POST: Random House Books
c/o Bookpost, PO Box 29, Douglas
Isle of Man, IM99 1BQ

BY FAX: 01624 670923

BY EMAIL: bookshop@enterprise.net

Cheques (payable to Bookpost) and credit cards accepted.

Prices and availability subject to change without notice.
Allow 28 days for delivery.
When placing your order, please mention if you do
not wish to receive any additional information.

www.rbooks.co.uk